The Role o [...] by Michael E. Lamb

Handbook of Behavioral Assessment [...] ny R. Ciminero, Karen S. Calhoun, and Henry E. Adams

Counseling and Psychotherapy: A Behavioral Approach by E. Lakin Phillips

Dimensions of Personality edited by Harvey London and John E. Exner, Jr.

The Mental Health Industry: A Cultural Phenomenon by Peter A. Magaro, Robert Gripp, David McDowell, and Ivan W. Miller III

Nonverbal Communication: The State of the Art by Robert G. Harper, Arthur N. Wiens, and Joseph D. Matarazzo

Alcoholism and Treatment by David J. Armor, J. Michael Polich, and Harriet B. Stambul

A Biodevelopmental Approach to Clinical Child Psychology: Cognitive Controls and Cognitive Control Theory by Sebastiano Santostefano

Handbook of Infant Development edited by Joy D. Osofsky

Understanding the Rape Victim: A Synthesis of Research Findings by Sedelle Katz and Mary Ann Mazur

Childhood Pathology and Later Adjustment: The Question of Prediction by Loretta K. Cass and Carolyn B. Thomas

Intelligent Testing with the WISC-R by Alan S. Kaufman

Adaptation in Schizophrenia: The Theory of Segmental Set by David Shakow

Psychotherapy: An Eclectic Approach by Sol L. Garfield

Handbook of Minimal Brain Dysfunctions edited by Herbert E. Rie and Ellen D. Rie

Handbook of Behavioral Interventions: A Clinical Guide edited by Alan Goldstein and Edna B. Foa

Art Psychotherapy by Harriet Wadeson

Handbook of Adolescent Psychology edited by Joseph Adelson

Psychotherapy Supervision: Theory, Research and Practice edited by Allen K. Hess

Psychology and Psychiatry in Courts and Corrections: Controversy and Change by Ellsworth A. Fersch, Jr.

Restricted Environmental Stimulation: Research and Clinical Applications by Peter Suedfeld

Personal Construct Psychology: Psychotherapy and Personality edited by Alvin W. Landfield and Larry M. Leitner

Mothers, Grandmothers, and Daughters: Personality and Child Care in Three-Generation Families by Bertram J. Cohler and Henry U. Grunebaum

Further Explorations in Personality edited by A.I. Rabin, Joel Aronoff, Andrew M. Barclay, and Robert A. Zucker

Hypnosis and Relaxation: Modern Verification of an Old Equation by William E. Edmonston, Jr.

Handbook of Clinical Behavior Therapy edited by Samuel M. Turner, Karen S. Calhoun, and Henry E. Adams

Handbook of Clinical Neuropsychology edited by Susan B. Filskov and Thomas J. Boll

The Course of Alcoholism: Four Years After Treatment by J. Michael Polich, David J. Armor, and Harriet B. Braiker

Handbook of Innovative Psychotherapies edited by Raymond J. Corsini

The Role of the Father in Child Development (Second Edition) edited by Michael E. Lamb

Behavioral Medicine: Clinical Applications by Susan S. Pinkerton, Howard Hughes, and W.W. Wenrich

Handbook for the Practice of Pediatric Psychology edited by June M. Tuma

Change Through Interaction: Social Psychological Processes of Counseling and Psychotherapy by Stanley R. Strong and Charles D. Claiborn

Drugs and Behavior (Second Edition) by Fred Leavitt

(continued on back)

The Dynamics of Art Psychotherapy

Harriet Wadeson, Ph.D., ATR
University of Illinois at Chicago

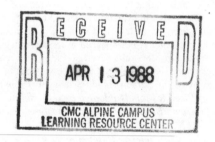
A WILEY-INTERSCIENCE PUBLICATION

JOHN WILEY & SONS

New York · Chichester · Brisbane · Toronto · Singapore

Library of Congress Cataloging in Publication Data:
Wadeson, Harriet, 1931–
   The dynamics of art psychotherapy.

   (Wiley series on personality processes)
   "A Wiley-Interscience publication."
   Includes bibliographies and indexes.
   1. Art therapy.   2. Psychotherapy.   I. Title.
II. Series.   [DNLM: 1. Art Therapy.   WM 450.5.A8 W121d]

RC489.A7W34   1986   616.89'1656   86-26710
ISBN 0-471-83137-9

Printed in the United States of America

10 9 8 7 6 5 4 3 2 1

To my many students
who have taught me so much

Series Preface

This series of books is addressed to behavioral scientists interested in the nature of human personality. Its scope should prove pertinent to personality theorists and researchers as well as to clinicians concerned with applying an understanding of personality processes to the amelioration of emotional difficulties in living. To this end, the series provides a scholarly integration of theoretical formulations, empirical data, and practical recommendations.

Six major aspects of studying and learning about human personality can be designated: personality theory, personality structure and dynamics, personality development, personality assessment, personality change, and personality adjustment. In exploring these aspects of personality, the books in the series discuss a number of distinct but related subject areas: the nature and implications of various theories of personality; personality characteristics that account for consistencies and variations in human behavior; the emergence of personality processes in children and adolescents; the use of interviewing and testing procedures to evaluate individual differences in personality; efforts to modify personality styles through psychotherapy, counseling, behavior, therapy, and other methods of influence; and patterns of abnormal personality functioning that impair individual competence.

IRVING B. WEINER

Fairleigh Dickinson University
Rutherford, New Jersey

v

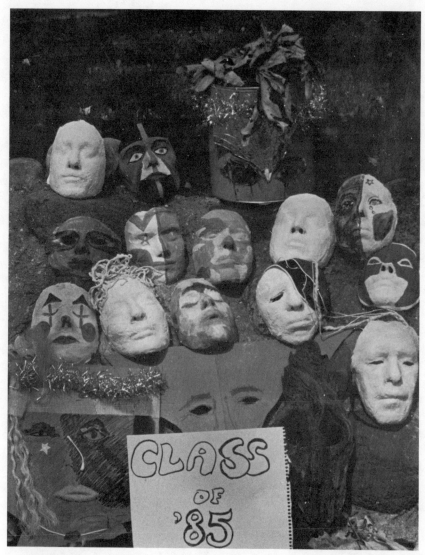

Figure 1. Masks made at University of Illinois first Art Therapy Summer Institute.

Preface

One who teaches learns. Having taught art therapy for 15 years and directed and developed art therapy graduate programs for the past eight years, I have had much opportunity for learning. In the dynamic interchange between student and teacher, ideas have germinated, matured, transformed, and led to new ideas and new connections. Vague understandings have become articulated. The questions never cease. The student is challenged to develop the self into an art therapist—one who integrates the worlds of art and human understanding to encourage creative self-expression accompanied by creative self-exploration. The art therapy teacher's continuing quest is to provide the most fertile soil to nourish students' growth.

It is from that soil that this book has grown. Whereas clients and patients had been my instructors for my previous book, *Art Psychotherapy* (1980), for this book I am indebted to my students. As my efforts to stimulate their thinking stimulated my own, we reached together for the ideas that have taken shape on these pages.

I wrote *Art Psychotherapy* to give form and integration to my clinical experience and because many asked for such a book. I have written *The Dynamics of Art Psychotherapy* to draw together the probings and reflections that have resulted from training art therapists. Simultaneously, the field has reached the stage in its development where it needs more penetrating perspectives. Much writing in art therapy has been descriptive. This has been important for a young profession. But now there is need to address with greater scrutiny the understandings that inform our efforts.

Whereas *Art Psychotherapy* illustrated work with diverse populations, this book attempts to explore the rationale behind the work, the principles that form the foundation of art therapists' efforts. There is a dynamic interchange between principles and practice, each informing the other. Art therapy hasn't grown the way one would build a house, by first

completing a firm foundation upon which the rest of the structure stands.
The more organic metaphor of a plant's growth fits better. Roots continue
to develop as the plant grows.

This book is a distillation of art therapy as I practice it, teach it, and
understand it. For its title I have used the term "Art Psychotherapy."
There are those whose work with patients in a treatment setting utilizes
art for recreational or artistic purposes. These activities are often designated art therapy. I use the term "Art Psychotherapy" to distinguish the
sort of art therapy I practice and teach from its use as a recreational or
occupational therapy activity. "Art psychotherapy," as the term suggests, is a mode of psychotherapy utilizing art. Its purpose is therapy, not
art, recreation, or a product-oriented activity. Throughout this book when
I refer to "art therapy," I hope it is clear that I mean the term in its
generic sense, rather than as differentiated from "art psychotherapy." In
most cases, the two are used interchangeably except where I especially
distinguish "art psychotherapy" from other practices also designated art
therapy.

The book is organized so that chapters and sections may be read either
singly or in sequence. With the former in mind, some topics are touched
upon in one chapter and developed more fully in another, particularly for
such issues as professional identity, transference, assessment—subjects
that are relevant to a number of aspects of the work. Some chapters
include basics to provide a framework for the more probing discussions
that follow, for example the information on art materials followed by their
transference ramifications. In general I have tried to address issues that I
believe are thought-provoking with foundation backgrounds included
only for elucidation of the more complex material. Most of the chapters
contain new viewpoints about which little or nothing has been written
previously. Some of the ideas may be controversial. It is my hope that
they will stimulate your thinking.

I wish this book could be received in the way a painting is viewed, by
taking it in all at once so that the full gestalt is immediately manifest. As a
book's content is sequential in progression, I have had to make some
difficult decisions in the organization of its content. Nevertheless, I wish
you could know about the Context of Art Therapy while you're reading
about the Phases in Art Therapy and understand the Elements of Art
Therapy while you're reading about The Art Therapist. Therefore, I hope
you will feel free to roam about the book and perhaps return to earlier
chapters after having read later ones.

I have tried to paint a balanced picture. The field of art therapy is
illuminated with strokes of brilliant colors; but it has its shadows as well.

This book presents some of the problems that beleaguer the profession as well as its considerable strengths.

As you read this volume, I hope you will be light on your feet in your understanding of the field as I have presented it, so that you will be able to shift balance gracefully to accommodate the changes that I may not have envisioned at the time of writing. My intention is to articulate ideas in order to create a response in you, the reader. I hope this book will cause you to pause and reflect, maybe to rethink some ideas you've had or to develop new ones out of the promptings this writing has urged. I would like nothing better than to create a dialogue. So if my thoughts stir any of your own, I would be most interested in hearing from you.

HARRIET WADESON

Chicago, Illinois
March 1987

Acknowledgments

Thanks to the colleagues and students who generously loaned their art-work and that of their clients for inclusion in this book. It has been great fun for me to photograph many of those who people my professional life. I'm grateful for the opportunity to present their liveliness in the illustrations here just as I have appreciated the opportunity to work with them as students and colleagues. I'm also grateful to those who supplied me with photographs they had taken. Pat Allen, Evadne McNeil, Ellen Sontag, Susan Johnson, and Joanne Ramsayer kindly read early drafts of the manuscript and gave me useful feedback and suggestions. My mother, Sophie Weisman, lovingly typed some of the early chapters. Robin Ukockis undertook most of the typing and, despite my indecipherable handwriting, remained cheerful throughout. Ungrateful acknowledgment goes to my four cats who walked over my papers, sat on them as I tried to read and write them, and generally did what they could to distract me from completing this book.

Contents

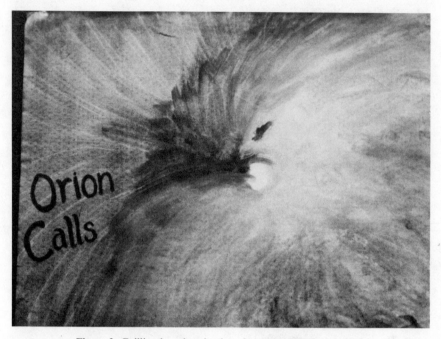

Figure 2. Brilliantly colored galaxy by manic atomic scientist.

INTRODUCTION

Art and Therapy, the Best of Both Worlds

Art therapy is not the addition of art-making to therapy nor the addition of therapy to art. It is a synthesis, a new entity, in the same way that water is not simply hydrogen plus oxygen. Although art therapy is both an art and therapy, it is more.

Expression in art stimulates fantasy, creativity, spontaneous unconscious imagery. It offers the possibility of creating a self-reflection, an image of oneself and one's world, from which it is possible to separate to gain distance. In this way the art object may provide a unique self-confrontation and perspective. Art-making may be an occasion for joy and fun as well as serious contemplation. Materials are manipulated to form beautiful, strange, bizarre, ugly, pleasing, amusing images.

The act of creating is a striving toward mastery. To view the work of one's own hands can be an exhilarating experience. It can also be frustrating when one feels discouraged in being unable to express visually what one has in mind. Nevertheless, the artist is in control to create whatever the imagination prompts. One may modify the world or create an entirely new world. In art-making, perhaps we come closer to being like a god/, goddess than in any other endeavor.

Whereas art-making can occur in solitude, therapy implies a relationship between at least two people, one of whom is the therapist and one the client. That partnership has been described in many ways, but the most fruitful descriptive term I have found is the "therapeutic alliance." An alliance implies a working together, rather than one person doing something to or for another.

The word "therapy" may connote sickness or pathology that needs to be fixed. It is an unfortunate connotation. Students, in particular, often feel they must do something. But therapy is a more subtle sort of stimulation.

Perhaps the analogy of gardening is applicable. The gardener cultivates

1

the soil to prepare a proper bed for growth, then weeds and waters during growth. But the gardener does not grow the seeds; the seeds do their own growing. Many patients and clients have never had favorable conditions for growth. The sunlight may have been blocked, the soil too acid, the water too scarce. Many people experience understanding and non-judgmental support in therapy such as they have never had before in their lives. Many find in themselves for the first time strengths and beauty that had been hidden. Many learn to trust and discover in the therapeutic garden that there is possibility for safety and others who are not weeds. Therapy at its best gives people what they should have come by naturally in their growing but which, unfortunately, so many have not received.

Art therapy is more than art used therapeutically or therapy to which art is added for further expressive possibilities. There is a very special sort of relationship that evolves through sharing of imagery. The internal world of images is a private one. Fantasy and creativity are stimulated as one tries to capture that world in the visible medium of art materials. Fleeting images, sometimes mysterious in their origins, pause on paper or in clay to be viewed and shared. It is the art therapist who prompts this way of bringing the inside out. And it is with the art therapist that a special sort of intimacy is created, an intimacy that allows another to see literally what is within and to witness the mysterious process of creation that art therapy is.

The self-expression and exploration, the creation of a world, that are part of art-making combine with the positive personal development fostered by the therapeutic alliance to form a new way of self-expression and discovery. From this unique engagement, a new kind of intimacy develops. This synthesis, rooted in imagistic connections and shared with one sensitive to this process, is the ineffable power of art therapy.

Elsewhere (Wadeson, 1980), I have written of the advantages art therapy offers and how I have used it with many populations. On the following pages I will try to detail what the art therapist actually does and why. I begin with who the art therapist is.

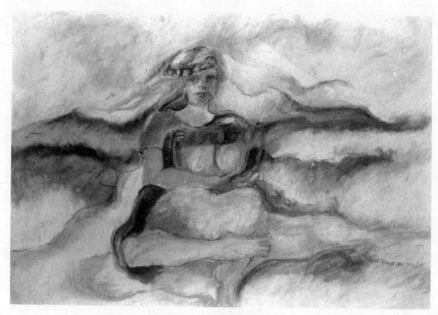

Figure 3. Portrait of the author by Anne Romig.

PART ONE

The Art Therapist

Art therapy is created by the art therapist in concert with her clients and patients. The unique qualities the art therapist brings to the work determines its nature. Like any work of art or other creative endeavor, the outcome of art therapy bears the imprint of its creator. As in artistic expression, an art therapy encounter is more than paints and brushes; it is the self that the artist puts into it. This section explores the self the art therapist brings to the work, encompassing therapeutic personality, theoretical approach, and professional identity.

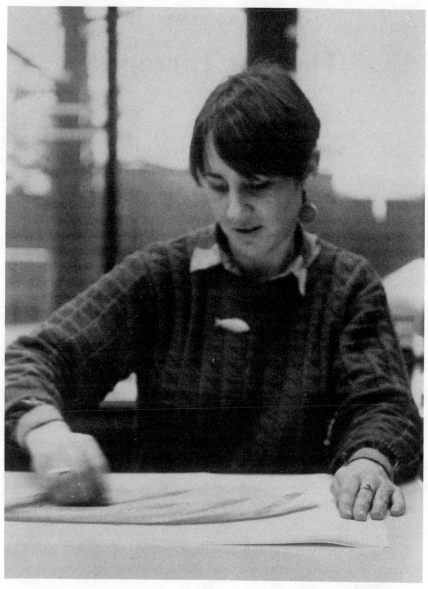

Figure 4. Art therapist Elizabeth Day is intent on creating her own art.

CHAPTER 1

The Art Therapist

The most likely way to discuss art therapy is by beginning with art-making (such as materials and methods), or with therapy (such as human development and pathology). But my belief is that the art therapy process begins with the art therapist. Some might argue that the art therapist isn't even necessary, that have used their own art-making experience and its creative exploration to further their personal growth without benefit of an art therapist. I would not disagree, and in fact I count myself among those who have grown significantly through self-exploration in creative self-expression. Nevertheless, when I discuss art therapy, I do not mean solitary artmaking. I am referring to a helping profession in which, by definition, art therapists are employed to work with others.

The art therapist is the constant in the equation. Her art materials, place of work, conditions of work, and clients may vary, but she is who she is.* And who she is determines the nature of the therapeutic interaction. But she is only a *relative* constant in this equation. Her work is dynamic, and she grows and adapts according to what she confronts. That process is described at length throughout this book.

But first let's take a look at who she is and what she brings to the art therapy experience. She brings with her no less than her total life experience. Although this is true for everyone in every situation, in psychotherapeutic work it makes a difference. For example, if I were a surgeon, it would be important that I know how to diagnose, to perform surgery, and to effect after-care. It probably wouldn't matter whether I was a parent or not. In performing psychotherapy, on the other hand, I must bring my total self to the relationship with my client. Having children effects my view of myself, of others, of the world, of life itself. It does not simply enable me to understand another parent's experience more empathically; it changes me in subtle and indirect ways that are of such complexity they can never be fully sorted through.

---

* Although the art therapist may be male or female, throughout this book I refer to her as female since this book is composed of my understandings, and I am female.

So the art therapist brings to each session her angry mother, her withdrawn father, her joy in her own creativity, the death of her dog, her warm smile, her love of mystery stories, her wish to get more exercise, or whatever experiences and traits make her who she is. As a result, no two therapists will ever do therapy in exactly the same way, even though their objectives and training may be almost identical. Each one's work will bear the imprint of her personality and her unique creativity.

PERSONALITY CHARACTERISTICS

Are there some life experiences and personality traits that auger well or poorly for the art therapist? I believe there are. Not everyone is well-suited for this sort of work. The personality characteristics I believe are propitious or unfavorable are difficult to delineate because they are not exact and there can be impressive exceptions. Therefore, I hope you will bear in mind that what follows is composed of generalizations, not necessarily subject to measurement or rigid adherence.

Positive Qualities

The first positive attribute is an obvious one—a caring and concern for others. Empirical research has demonstrated that those therapists found most helpful by their patients received high ratings in "accurate empathy, nonpossessive warmth, and genuineness." Other factors, such as theoretical approach or method of therapy were not statistically significant (Yalom, 1975, pp. 45, 46).

Concern or caring for others may not be as simple or as obvious as it seems at first glance. When my students begin their training, I ask them why they want to be art therapists. Many respond, "Because I want to help others." They sound altruistic. I hope they are not. The practice of therapy requires the total presence of the therapist; it is so much more than a skill; the therapist brings her creativity and vulnerability to every therapeutic encounter. Therefore, if her heart and soul are not in her work, it is not likely to be very good work. If she is not getting something out of the work for herself, she is probably burned out and should move on to other enterprises.

I ask my students to look beyond their wish to help others in order to try to understand what they derive personally from such an experience. Usually, they come to recognize their own needs for intimacy, for stimulation (artistic and otherwise), for power, and for meaningful impact on others so that they are valued and experienced as important. Such needs might be seen as exploitative of the patient. After all, most people don't seek therapy in order to provide intimacy and status for their therapist.

The pivotal point is self-awareness. When the patient's needs and the therapist's needs are synergistic, there is no problem. When the therapist is aware that she is tempted to use the patient for her own gratification, then she can check herself. If she doesn't even know her own needs, this sort of self-monitoring becomes impossible.

For example, I had a client who would look to me for "the word from on high." She would be so appreciative every time I spouted a little lesson in life and gaze at me with such rapt attention, that from time to time I found myself giving her little speeches. On reflection, I realized that what she needed was to take more responsibility and not look to me for answers. It was my grandiosity that was playing into her dependency.

The point I am trying to make is two-fold. First, therapists need personal gratification to participate fully in the demanding therapeutic process. If we had no personal needs gratified by the work, it would become personally meaningless. Second, it is essential to be aware of what our needs are so that we don't gratify them at our clients' expense. And as an aside, I hope the foregoing example illustrates that it is not fatal to make small mistakes as I did with my overly-dependent client. The lack of self-awareness that is exploitative is pervasive use of the client to satisfy intimacy, power, control, and self-aggrandizement needs.

Having strayed a bit from positive personality characteristics of the art therapist, let us return to one already discussed, but not specifically identified: self-awareness. Since therapy exists in the context of the therapeutic relationship, it is impossible for the therapist to understand what her client is experiencing if she does not have a perspective on the relationship between herself and her client. In order to understand that relationship, she must be able to process her own reactions. Some therapists have been known to view their clients as through a microscope, putting themselves in the role of observer without recognition of their own strong influence on the therapeutic process. Because therapy is an interaction, the therapist cannot see it fully if she is blind to her side of the equation.

For example, I noticed that at times during sessions my eyes went out of focus. I came to realize that this was a reaction to distancing measures the client was instigating. Once I recognized my own distancing response, I was able to comment on it to the client and question what was going on between us. This, of course, brought us back in touch with one another to explore our relationship and the immediate events in the therapy together. Without my reflection on myself, we probably would have remained out of touch during the session.

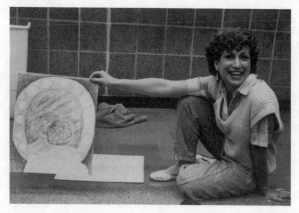

Figure 5. Diane Evans, art therapy student, displaying her drawing of herself confronting a mirror in her striving for self-awareness.

Self-awareness is not an established characteristic, but rather an ongoing, life-long refinement of sensitivity to one's own processes. So in determining whether one would become an art therapist, the inclination toward self-awareness should be considered. It is helpful for therapists to be persons who have grappled with existential questions of life and death because these form a basis for how one lives, the essential issue for therapy. Some people enjoy introspection. It's not everyone's cup of tea. And then there are those who are so heavily defended that it would take years of work for them to peel the layers of denial from their eyes.

Another important characteristic is openness. It is essential to understand the client's view of the world. Although we each have our own belief system and our own values, it is necessary to transcend them in order to try to see the client's world through the client's eyes. Of course, we cannot and should not put aside our own beliefs, but we can try to shift frames of reference in order to understand our clients' experience. Those who are not open to this mode of thought will probably have difficulty doing effective therapy.

For example, if you believe abortion is a sin and your client is planning to have one, how do you react? If your client believes he* is being poisoned by the devil, do you merely label him paranoid or try to imagine what he is experiencing? I worked with a manic-depressive man who was

* Although the client (or patient) could be male or female, throughout this book I refer to him as male to distinguish him from the art therapist for whom the female pronoun is used.

a "wheeler-dealer," constantly dropping names and trying to have contact with prominent people. His world and value system were very different from mine, but it was important for me to understand the dimensions of his world as he had structured it. I tried to imagine what it must have been like for him, rather than to analyze and judge him.

Some belief systems do not allow for others. For example, I interviewed an applicant for art therapy graduate training who seemed a promising candidate in most respects. The problem was that she was a *born-again* Christian whose intention was to use art therapy to "save souls." I recommended that she pursue pastoral counseling instead. Though well-intentioned, her integrity as a prospective art therapist was questionable. Her religious beliefs taught her that the highest form of service was to "save" others. Some people do not want that sort of "salvation." I believe it is imperative for therapists to respect and encourage their clients' thoughtful life decisions.

A positive attribute difficult to describe is intelligence. We don't even know what it is, and no doubt, there are many kinds. Since therapy is the sort of work for which there are no pat formulas, the therapist is required to make decisions minute by minute, often with no time to deliberate. This sort of rapid reacting, as well as the slower conceptualizations necessary in putting together the pieces of the client's complex personal puzzle, require intelligence. It isn't enough, therefore, for the art therapist to be warm and well-meaning, though such people can provide significant nurturing. To make some kind of sense of it all requires intelligence.

But what about therapists who appear to have an intuitive grasp of the work? I had a student who would joke that she had no left brain, that she operated totally out of her right brain. I believe that what we call intuition is not mysterious or magical, but is based on a special kind of learning and intelligence. Often what may be seen as an intuitive reaction or understanding derives from synthesizing that is integrated so rapidly or through unidentified channels so that the process is indiscernible, in contrast to the more familiar steps of inductive or deductive analytical reasoning.

Related to intelligence is the ability for self-direction. Because therapy cannot be reduced to learned routines, the therapist must write her own script. The work often benefits from her inventiveness as well.

Intelligence and inventiveness are components of creativity. Hopefully, the therapeutic alliance is a creative relationship in which the therapist relates in ways that may be new in the client's experience. The goal is for the client to partake of that creativity in developing more creative solutions to living. Because no two people are the same, each client provides the therapist with a unique challenge to her creativity in therapy.

Up to this point, all the attributes described apply to many kinds of therapists, not specifically to art therapists. Although creativity also applies to all therapists, it has special meaning for art therapists. Creative image-making is the core of art therapy and that which distinguishes it from other modes of therapy. Art expression is a creative endeavor even when it is more process than product-oriented, as in art therapy. Therefore, the art therapist has a special relationship to the creative as she encourages her clients to dip into their unconscious, their fantasies, dreams, experiences, perspectives, to exercise their spontaniety in the creating of their art expressions. If she has not developed her own creativity, it is not likely that she will be successful in encouraging others to do so.

It is important, therefore, that in addition to approaching life creatively, as is desirable in all therapists, for the art therapist to have experienced her own creative art expression for self-understanding and personal growth. Although this experience is a part of a necessary background rather than a personality characteristic, it is mentioned here because it is an operational manifestation of her creativity. In other words, the art therapist is one whose creativity has led her to self-development through her own art expression. The important aspect is not the production of works of high artistic merit. In fact, an over-concern with the formal properties of successful art may even get in the way of awareness of its personal dimensions. This awareness and the advancement of self-knowledge and growth through the synthesizing functions of art-making constitute the significance of an art background for the practice of art therapy. It is evident that an art therapist who believes in her work would encourage art expression not only for her clients but for herself as well.

Creativity is a complex characteristic with many aspects. One of them worth mentioning is playfulness. The spontaneity of the art experience and the freedom to represent anything in any way offers the possibility of fun. Certainly the art therapist should be able to make the most of this potentiality, particularly for patients whose lives or approaches to life may otherwise be quite grim. The freedom to be playful when it is helpful is a most desirable attribute.

Empathy and high motivation are expected positive attributes. I have left them for last because I would like to discuss them in a special way, in the context of "the wounded healer."

Empathy grows out of personal experience. The only way I can connect with my client's feelings of loneliness is through my own experience of loneliness. Although my life situation may be very different from his, there is a commonality of human emotions we have shared. It isn't by analyzing his condition as an outside observer that I come to know him empathically, but rather by recognizing my feelings of anger, helplessness, fear, or whatever emotions he is experiencing. The ability to empathize, to join with the client on the feeling level, is necessary in building the therapeutic relationship.

The concept of "the wounded healer" is related to the foundations of empathy. It is not the unscathed individual who has managed a life relatively free of problems that makes the best healer, but rather one who has faced life's viccissitudes, received its wounds, and survived. She can draw on those life experiences to understand and help her clients and patients face and deal with life. A therapist who has suffered little in life may be less sensitive to the suffering of others.*

In addition to the personal gratifications therapists may derive from helping others, motivation may be embodied in "the wounded healer" position. The long and painful process of healing oneself may be fostered by similar work with others. Some people who turn inwards with sensitivity to their own hurts enter the therapeutic professions as part of their own self-healing. Many of my art therapy students give as a reason for wanting to become an art therapist the wish to understand themselves more fully. There is no question that we learn much about ourselves and about life from our intimate work with our clients.

These and many other interpersonal characteristics, such as an ease in relating to others, social skills, the ability to inspire confidence, articulateness, and so forth, we assume to be desirable aspects of the therapist's make-up. A continuing stretching in personal and professional development is also assumed to be characteristic of the responsible professional. Obviously, a significant lack of many of these attributes would bode poorly for the likelihood of positive professional development. Although it may seem that the professional I am describing would be close to saintliness, I hope it is clear that it is her humanness, not her perfection, that brings her close to those who seek her help. The positive attributes I have described are directions rather than perfections.

THEORETICAL ORIENTATION

The field of art therapy has not developed a theoretical foundation to inform its application. Unlike psychoanalysis, Jungian analytical psychology, gestalt therapy, transactional analysis, or even behavior modifica-

* See Guggenbuhl-Craig (1971) for a more thorough discussion of "the wounded healer."

tion, art therapy does not postulate a paradigm of human development or psychic organization. We have no concepts comparable to Freud's Id, Jung's shadow, the child of transactional analysis, the top-dog of gestalt therapy, the stimulus of behavior modification, or comparable concepts used in other approaches. Like other expressive therapies, art therapy recognizes the importance of creativity but advances no notions of how humans develop and function. Art therapists tend to borrow from the more established disciplines. Therefore, some art therapists work from a foundation in psychoanalytic theory, some are Jungians, and so forth.

Professional identity, therefore, may embody a theoretical orientation as well as the practice of art therapy. The issue of identity may be more complex than it initially appears. Often, art therapists work in isolation from other art therapists. Few treatment teams employ more than one art therapist, and it is not uncommon for the art therapist to find herself the facility's sole art therapy practitioner. Therefore, in addition to being bereft of art therapy theory, she is likely to lack art therapy models or even someone from her discipline with whom to share ideas or ask questions. Particularly for those just starting out, the need for professional identity is strong, and the more readily available models in both theoretical foundation and in professional practitioners may fill the vacuum.

Although there is much to learn from carefully developed theories and experienced practitioners (such as psychiatrists, psychologists, social workers), the art therapist may relinquish creative potentialities in art therapy by too readily adopting a fully developed paradigm. Because art therapy is more than a technique, much can be gained from evolving understandings from its unique processes. Psychological theories have tended to germinate from practice. Freud and Jung did not complete their theories and then go into practice. Rather, the evolution of their concepts derived from observations from their ongoing work in conjunction with deep introspection.

Almost by definition, art therapists are creative people. Yet, being a young profession, we have tended to look to the more mature mental health disciplines for both theory and methods of practice. I believe we should consider seriously the following admonishment from Jung:

I can only hope and wish that no one becomes "Jungian" . . . I proclaim no cut-and-dried doctrine and abhor 'blind adherents.' I leave everyone free to deal with the facts in his own way, since I also claim this freedom for myself." (Goldenberg, 1979) (no source given for quote).

In our present stage of development, there are art therapists who are Freudians, Jungians, and so forth. There are also psychiatrists, psychologists, social workers, nurses, occupational and recreational therapists of various theoretical persuasions who use art in their work with patients. What is needed, I believe, is the application of art therapists' creativity to the understanding and evolution of our own profession.

Consequently, I consider it important for art therapists to gain a background in all the major theories of psychic development and organization rather than the "narrow adherence" Jung abhorred. We must recognize that these concepts are ways of structuring understanding rather than ultimate truths. The complexity of the human psyche can be viewed from many vantage points, all of which may be "correct." Each has its limitations as well. Of course, one's work is less confusing if it can be understood from the perspective of one internally consistent paradigm.

The problem, however, is as Jung stated it. He developed an approach that grew out of his unique experience. Art therapy is a creative enterprise in its central activity of image creation, the creative exploration of the images, and the unique therapeutic relationship that becomes established. Because the therapist brings to each therapeutic encounter her individual life experience, her view must be her own. Therefore, fundamental to what I believe art therapy is about is the necessity for individual synthesizing of theory. I see this as a dynamic process in which the art therapist continues to learn and develop. Instead of finding "the true word," she is open to learning from various paradigms which help her to understand her own experience. But that experience is paramount.

For example, early in my career when I was working at the National Institute of Mental Health in the National Institutes of Health's Clinical Center in Bethedsa, Maryland, Stanley, a red-headed adolescent, was depicted by another art therapy group member as addicted to coca-cola, Figure 6. Stanley was given to outbursts of temper, and in fact during one group art therapy session, smashed the coke bottle he always brought to the group art therapy session. His psychiatrist diagnosed him as anally fixated with oral dependency needs. This didn't have much meaning for me. I saw Stanley as not so different from other adolescents I had known who were struggling with identity problems. He frequently acted pompous in a way that appeared an attempt to cover his feelings of inadequacy. About Figure 6, he said, "After all, it's one of my philosophies of life that life without one vice is no life at all . . . so far cokes are my only vice." The point I am trying to make is that a notion of anal or oral fixation was not helpful to me in understanding Stanley. Issues of power, control, and self-worth were helpful. Being new to the world of mental health, I related to him on the basis of my experience rather than on theories I did not understand. Now, over two decades later, I would recommend the same approach to beginning professionals.

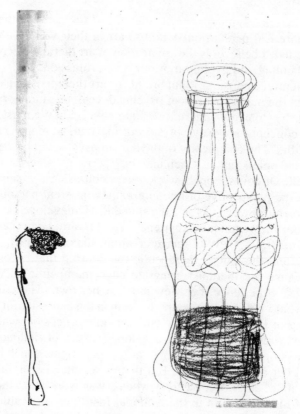

Figure 6. Hospitalized adolescent's picture of a fellow patient.

When I was starting out I was reading psychoanalytic theory and working in a psychoanalytically-oriented research and treatment program. But it seemed to me that the central issue for most of my patients was not conflict between basic drives and socialization, although this issue was not irrelevant for them. The more significant problem appeared to be their feelings about themselves, although, of course, the conflict between drives and socialization certainly effects feelings about the self. Nevertheless, it was more meaningful to me to question how my patients viewed themselves and their world than to conceptualize basic drives.

I have seen what Jung described as ''narrow adherence'' to theory interfere with a more creative approach to processing experience and valuing one's own wisdom. What I am suggesting is not that art therapists abandon theory, but rather that we synthesize from various possibilities for understanding that which is congruent with our own life experiences and views, as well as our clinical observations. This then becomes both an active and receptive process. It requires creativity in sorting and fitting together.

Needless to say, there are many art therapists who do excellent work in the framework of a particular theory they have found congenial to their own personal philosophy. I am only suggesting that the selection of theoretical foundations be a thoughtful one, rather than the "narrow adherence" Jung abhorred.

I will close this section with my favorite example of the limiting of understanding that may result from "narrow adherence" to theory. In a presentation I was giving to a hospital staff, the senior psychiatrist was particularly interested in the delusion drawn by Vickie, a young woman diagnosed acute schizophrenic. Just prior to entering the hospital she repeatedly experienced being stalked in a back alley by a "big black man, a killer," Figure 7. The senior psychiatrist became quite excited about his interpretation of the picture. Influenced by his classical psychoanalytic training, he was oriented toward sexual symbolism and saw the figure as a penis within the vaginal canal. From that point of view a therapist might be intent on digging for unconscious sexual conflict and neglect other important aspects of this drawing for the patient. Vickie was a withdrawn young woman who had spent the several months prior to hospitalization almost completely alone shut in her apartment. Her delusion was a confusing experience in which she did not know which parts were real and which weren't. By drawing it she was able to begin to make some sense out of this experience, and defuse some of the terror it held for her. More importantly, by sharing it with me she could undercut the isolation in which she had been enveloped for many months. No doubt the delusion and the drawing expressed significant unconscious processes as well. What they were was impossible to know at that time—which brings me to a final point.

Theory enables us to know. Sometimes it is better not to know. When there is little data, it is better to be open to possibilities rather than to nail down a conclusion. Time and again I have heard staff conference presentations of newly admitted patients that are told in nice neat stories with conclusive interpretations of the patients' dynamics. Human functioning is much too complex for simple interpretations. Uncertainty breeds anxiety. So there is a tendency to come to closure with a complete dynamic picture based on a consistent theory. I am pleased by Frank Barron's study that demonstrates that a characteristic of creative people is a toler-

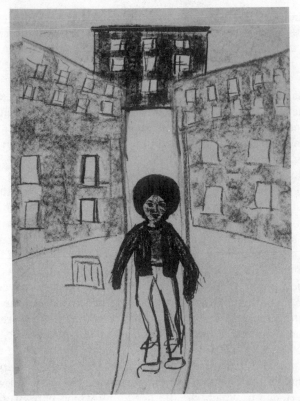

Figure 7. Delusion of a "big black man, a killer" stalking a schizophrenic young woman.

ance for ambiguity without a need to come to premature closure (Barron, 1968a and 1968b).

Hopefully, as the field of art therapy continues to develop, its potential for increasing our understanding of ourselves and other humans will lead to articulations from which we can learn. Although this book in no way attempts the major enterprise of forming an art therapy theory, my hope is that it provides a stepping stone along the way to a further realization of what we are doing and why we are doing it.

ARTIST/THERAPIST/ART THERAPIST

Issues of professional identity have been touched upon in the preceding pages in reference to theoretical orientation. Although members of various mental health disciplines may identify themselves as Jungians, gestalt therapists, and so forth, unique to the art therapy profession is the identification of artist.

Artist

What does it mean to be an artist? Does it mean that you make art? Does it mean that at one time you made art? Does it mean that you exhibit? Or is it a state of mind? Many art therapists come to art therapy from the world of art. Some studied art education. Some, but not all, have been exhibiting artists. Many have found that art therapy training and practice have been so demanding that they have little time for their own art. Some are faced with difficult choices. There are hardly any art therapists who have not been artists in one way or another. But it appears that the field is divided into those who continue to make art and give that activity a central position in their lives and those who no longer make art, having replaced it with art therapy, or who make art less frequently, giving it only a peripheral position in their lives.*

For many whose art-making is an important part of their lives, the identity of artist is a significant one. Some claim that it is necessary to be an artist with an artist's personal relationship to the creative process to be an art therapist.

The identity of artist trails behind it colorful connotations. Artists are stereotyped as temperamental, idiosyncratic sometimes to the point of eccentricity, independent, and self-directed. There are legends of those who sacrificed human relationships, material possessions, and comforts "for the sake of their art." Surely these romantic notions are extreme. Nevertheless, the independence and self-direction characteristic of the artist often lead others to expect that he or she will not necessarily conform to convention. Art therapists sometimes find that others with whom they work are receptive to their different way of working because there is a tolerance for an artist's individuality. The artist who prizes his or her creativity may be inclined to think independently and to apply creativity to the art therapy process.

On the negative side, artists sometimes surround their art with an aura of preciousness. I have witnessed artists fearful of discussion of their work lest in some way it might be destroyed or trivialized by words. This fear is difficult for me to understand. The art remains regardless of what is

---

* See *Design for Arts in Education*, September/October, 1984, for an issue devoted to Controversy, Artist or Therapist?

said. If its meaning or expression is significant to its creator, this too remains intact even if another fails to understand.

To return to the question implied but not answered, does an art therapist need to be an artist? I do not know the answer. As mentioned previously, I find it necessary for an art therapist to have had considerable experience in the process of self-expression and self-exploration through art-making in order to encourage others and to understand their process in this activity. I believe this involves a considerable portion of one's life, not simply a weekend workshop or even a semester course.

My art background has been varied. I have had fertile periods and droughts. These have been influenced by the many other things that were going on in my life. I have exhibited, won awards for my art, and been paralyzed in art expression for long periods of time. I have turned to other creative expressions such as short story, poetry, and play-writing. Despite many vicissitudes, I believe I have always retained my connection to the creative. There has been no period in my life in which I've lost the joy in my own creativity.

This last recognition is the key to my view of the art experience. Most artists I know refer to their art as their "work." If my art-making were work, I wouldn't do it. It is my play. It is this spirit of art that I bring to art therapy. I'm not sure how to define "artist" or whether one needs to be one to be an art therapist. I don't even know if delight in the creative process is essential. But I write these words having just spent most of the day painting an inner self-portrait and know that this painting and my art therapy work feed each other. As I stated earlier, the practice of art therapy is so individualized, I cannot say that what is a part of the self I bring to art therapy is necessary for another.

Therapist

Identification as a therapist does not parallel the ambiguity of "artist." The job of the art therapist is to provide therapy. In the term "art therapy," "therapy" is the noun and "art" an adjective—a descriptive modifier identifying the kind of therapy the term connotes. To my mind, there is no question that the art therapist is a therapist with all the training in human understanding and all the responsibility that this serious vocation requires.

Before art therapy developed into a recognized, respected discipline, artists volunteered their services in mental hospitals. Some were employed to provide art classes for the patients. For many patients, the opportunity to make art with a teacher sensitive to their needs became a therapeutic experience. But a therapeutic experience does not make therapy. Many people who are interested in others and who are nurturing by nature can relate to those in need with delicacy and compassion. The responsibility undertaken by a therapist is a special kind of commitment that goes beyond the efforts of a caring teacher. The therapeutic commitment will be discussed further in other sections of this book, but one important distinction deserves mention here. An artist is likely to be more product-oriented since his or her efforts are directed toward the production of high quality art. The therapist, on the other hand, is working for the patient's positive development, regardless of what sort of art expression the patient may produce.

Chapter 12 explores the approaches of "art as therapy" and "art psychotherapy." But for now I would like to raise a problem of definition. An art therapist with a strong artist identity who attaches a great deal of importance to the quality of the client's art productions may actually be functioning more like a sensitive art teacher than an art therapist. The important distinction is that the art therapist is a *therapist* in relation to her clients, not an artist or a teacher. That she uses art and often educates do not make her other than, first and foremost, a therapist.

Art Therapist

What it means to be an art therapist is what the rest of this book is about. But for the purposes of definition, an art therapist uses the process of art expression and its exploration to effect her clients' positive growth and the amelioration of their suffering. How this is done is detailed throughout this book.

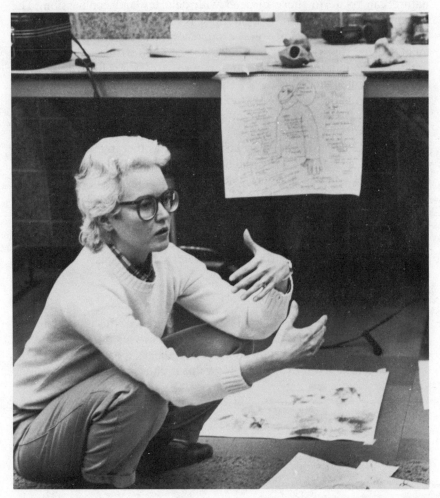

Figure 8. Discussion of one's art is an important part of the art therapy process, as illustrated here by Deborah Behnke-Marthaler.

PART TWO

Elements of Art Therapy

The actual doing of art therapy encompasses a number of elements. First, the stage must be set in creating an environment, selecting art materials, establishing a structure. Next there is the important step of encouraging the art expression. How the art therapist understands art expression is an area of professional controversy, assumptions, and neglect. A chapter of this section delineates a detailed perspective. Relating to clients and patients through and around their art expressions in order to promote their awareness and growth is one of the art therapists' most crucial areas of expertise. Finally, a chapter on group art therapy is included to discuss a prevalent mode of working for which scant training is offered and about which little has been written.

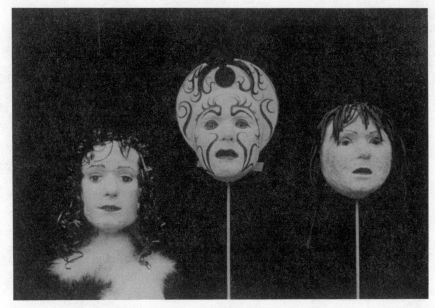

Figure 9. Self-portrait masks by Gilda Moreno.

CHAPTER 2

Structure, Environment, and Materials

Since the process of art therapy involves creating a product, logistical considerations of materials and workspace are more prominent than in many other modes of therapy. Before examining what happens in art psychotherapy, it is necessary to understand these important logistical and structural foundations of the work. Although it may seem as though all that is needed are a few art supplies and a place to work, in actuality the influence of session structure, workspace, and materials can be significant. These are the background elements of the work that help shape its evolution.

STRUCTURING ART THERAPY

Structure includes materials and space as well as the organization of the whole art therapy process. It begins with the manner in which people come to art therapy, by referral, self-selection, or as part of a facility's regular routine. The many aspects of time are especially significant in structure: length of sessions, frequency, and duration of the art therapy treatment regimen.

Time

Decisions about time are not made arbitrarily but with client needs and capacities and the total treatment framework in mind. Because the art therapist knows better than anyone else what is involved in the art-making and art-exploration process, it is she who should organize the art therapy schedule rather than its being imposed by other staff members.

A part of this organization is the structuring of both art-making and discussion time. In art therapy sessions for individuals, there can be much flexibility. Group time organization is more complicated and is discussed in Chapter 6.

If an art therapist is working in a short-term facility, she may need to have frequent sessions, perhaps every day, in order to establish a relationship in an abbreviated time period. If patients are disruptive or have poor attention spans, sessions may have to be short. Decisions regarding amount of time for art-making and exploring the finished piece should be based on patient needs. These may change over time, so flexibility is useful.

Consistency and continuity are important considerations in scheduling. Art therapy becomes an expectable process when there are specific and consistent meeting times that the patients can count on. Scheduling sessions catch-as-catch-can is disruptive to patients. On the other hand, an art therapist may wish to have open time available if a patient wants a session at a particular moment to meet immediate needs. In order for the process to be one that builds, scheduling should encourage continuity. It's difficult to build continuity if sessions are more than a week apart.

Many frameworks are possible: brief sessions, one or two hour sessions, all day or weekend workshops, and an open studio structure where patients can come and go as they please. The most widely used time frame is the hour session for individuals and one and a half to two hours for groups and families.

Sometimes I have scheduled sessions at particular times for particular purposes. At NIH there were occasions when I scheduled art therapy in the hour before the patient was to meet with his psychiatrist. This way the material stimulated by the art expression could be processed further in the psychiatric session. Sometimes I scheduled art therapy directly after verbal group therapy so that a patient could use the art to release feelings that may have been aroused in group. In doing evaluation work, my NIH sessions were sometimes arranged in accordance with certain medication regimens. In working with suicidal patients, I made a point of seeing them as soon as possible after a suicide attempt.

The open studio as a very loosely structured art therapy format is appropriate for certain purposes. Those invested in art-making can have access to materials and work space to use within each one's own time frame. If a therapeutic relationship is to be established, the art therapist must engage with patients around this activity. An open studio may be useful under other conditions as well. Some populations, such as emotionally disturbed children or adolescents, may need a place to come when needed where they can vent feelings or make projects. An art therapist may combine an open studio schedule with designated individual and group meetings.

Having discussed a few of the many variations art therapy structuring can take, I would like to emphasize that these arrangements are made with a great deal of thought. The art therapist devises a structure based on the goals, possibilities, and limitations of her work. Too often an art therapist may be pressured to fit her schedule into the institution's existing pattern rather than creating what may be a more facilitating or innovative framework. Obviously, she must work in concert with the treatment program of which she is a part or in consideration of clients' work or school schedules if they are out-patients. But I would recommend that she look first at what is needed, then consider what is possible. All too often we feel locked into a treatment or educational system that might benefit from modification. Although structure may seem to be a relatively mundane aspect of the art therapist's work, it is an important area to which she can apply her creativity to further the art therapy process.

Art Activities

In addition to the use of space, time, and materials, structure refers as well to the actual activity of art therapy. Is there an assigned task or does the client make the choices? Many factors influence the art therapist's decisions around more or less structure in the form of specific activities. Conditions under which an art therapist would structure a particular task include the gathering of specific information, attainment of a particular goal, or patient needs.

Gathering Information

Gathering of information is important for such purposes as assessment and treatment planning (including history taking) and research. The art therapist is not limited to the usual assessment methods of a verbal interview, but can gain much information through images. Frequently, I ask clients to draw a picture of their family of origin (Figure 10) and learn much through such elements as size of figures, placement of the figures, the surroundings or activities of family members shown, and their various characteristics that are depicted. A further assessment device is a representation of the precipitating conditions for treatment, such as a suicide attempt, drug problem, feelings of despair, and so forth. Requesting a self-image can also be useful in assessment, as perception of self is at the core of one's dynamics. (Assessment is discussed in greater detail in Chapter 7.)

For research purposes one may structure a session to gather information one is studying. For example, when I was studying suicide I asked suicidal patients to make pictures of their suicidal feelings. (See Wadeson, 1971b and 1975). When I was studying the phenomenology of acute schiz-

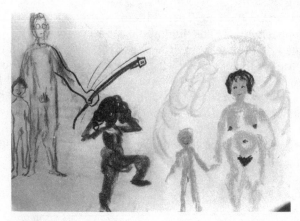

Figure 10. Family of origin by a woman who shows her anger in the dark figure (red) as she is beaten by her father and her brother pairs with each parent.

ophrenia, I asked patients to draw pictures of their psychiatric illness and hallucinations and delusions experienced. (See Wadeson and Carpenter, 1973, 1974 and 1976). When I was studying the marital relationship in manic-depressive psychosis, I asked couples to draw abstract pictures of their marital relationship and to make changes on one another's self-portraits (Figure 11). (See Wadeson and Fitzgerald, 1971). In utilizing specific tasks for research, it is important to inform the patients of the purpose of the exercises and to request their cooperation, rather than to give the impression that the activities are part of their treatment. Often, as with examples I have cited, the tasks served treatment functions as well. Nevertheless, since the structure of research design is usually fairly rigid in order to keep conditions constant from one patient to the next, it is necessary to explain the rationale. Also, if governed by treatment consid-erations only, the art therapist would probably structure the sessions differently, even if using some of the same exercises; therefore it would be a pretense to give an incorrect impression. Finally, it is usually neces-sary to obtain written consent for use of the art for presentation or publi-cation purposes.

Tasks for Treatment Goals

An art therapist might suggest a task to attain a specific treatment goal, such as a group mural to foster interaction, representations of feelings to enhance feeling awareness, depiction of a particular problematic experi-ence to gain perspective and understanding of it, drawings of fantasies to stimulate imagination and deal with wishes and fears, and so forth. The possibilities are limitless.

Conditions of Treatment

Finally, there may be conditions where more structure is beneficial. In short-term hospitalization, there is usually so little opportunity to work with clients that goals may have to be specific and limited. Often the appropriate goal would be dealing with the feelings about being hospitalized. If one is working in a group, there is also benefit for patients to be sharing such feelings. So a picture of these feelings may facilitate both a ventilation and processing of such feelings as well as some experience of universality and less isolation by sharing these images. The latter is often accomplished more readily with the added dimension of seeing others' images, rather than through talking alone, where some individuals are likely to be reticent (more about this in Chapter 6). If there has been a disruptive event of considerable influence, such as the suicide of a patient on the ward, the arrival of a new ward director, or a consequential change

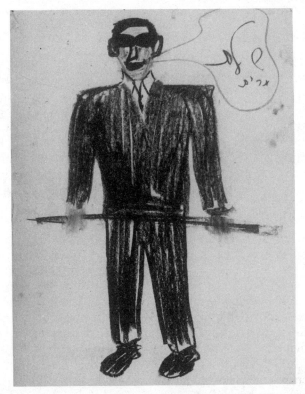

Figure 11. Self-portrait given to spouse. This man's schizophrenic wife added sunglasses, cane, the balloon coming out of his mouth, broadened his shoulders, and smeared his hands.

in the facility's policy, the art therapist might suggest that patients examine the event through the artwork.

Client Needs

Of a similar nature are events in the client's life that the art therapist would suggest be processed through art-making. The art therapist should be sensitive to the client's needs in these instances. For example, if a client is talking about a difficult experience or unpleasant feeling, the art therapist might suggest exploring that experience or feeling through the art. Nevertheless, it is also important that the art therapist be sensitive to a client's need to talk and not interrupt that flow with a suggestion to make art until art-making would be beneficial. At times the discussion of artwork might lead the art therapist to suggest that the elaboration of the reactions that come up for the client be explored by making a second art expression. Such a suggestion from the art therapist might be facilitating of both catharsis and insight.

Unstructured Art Activity

More important than the reasons for an art therapist providing a specific structured art activity, are the reasons for her not to do so. All too often art therapists feel they must do something. Some don't trust the process sufficiently to believe that through the facilitating means of image-making, in an encouraging environment and trusting relationship what needs to surface will. Generally, the art therapist does not have to push. Except in the circumstances just described, I do not suggest anything to my clients, but simply wait attentively for what they bring forth. For the most part, then, they do whatever they want. Even the most minimal drawing can be a vehicle of expression.

What I think is the most deleterious effect of over-structured art therapy is the insensitive imposition of irrelevant activity. This can happen when an art therapist decides in advance that on Tuesday she will ask her art therapy group to make pictures of a childhood fantasy. Perhaps on Monday a very frightening patient was admitted to the ward and the individuals in the group are caught up in their reactions to him. Her plan would be irrelevant and insensitive to current feelings. Sometimes an art therapist may learn a new technique at a workshop and be eager to try it out. It is important that she wait for an appropriate opportunity, rather than be guided by her own needs instead of those of her clients.

I try to encourage clients to be as responsible as possible for recognizing their own needs and finding ways of satisfying them. Therefore, I encourage them to devise their own structure for art activity, to decide, for example, that it might be useful to draw their parents' relationship or last night's dream or their anger or simply pound clay or whatever. I encourage them to know that although I might be able to provide some facilitating suggestions that they would not have thought of, in the long run they know themselves best and are best equipped to discover what they need. Therefore, if I make a suggestion and the client demurs, I might ask what he thinks would work better. If the refusal seems to result from resistance, on the other hand, then I try to explore with the client what might be getting in the way.

Sensitivity and Creativity in Structuring Art Therapy

Sensitivity and creativity, as in so many aspects of art therapy, are important in determining structure of art activity. Reacting out of her sensitivity to her clients' needs, the art therapist uses her creativity to develop a structure (or lack of it) of art-making that will advance the therapeutic process. The best art activities are often the most simple. Putting an event, feeling, fantasy, or dream into a picture or sculpture can be enormously releasing and illuminating. Too often art therapists grab for proven recipes other art therapists have designed, rather than responding to the situation at hand with a facilitating structure. I believe art therapists need to be responsive creatively rather than to store a repertoire of "techniques." In the training program I direct students learn few such techniques. They are encouraged to develop their own techniques or to refine those originated by others to meet the particular situations they encounter. This sort of creativity, like sensitivity in clinical judgement and refinement of self-awareness, is a part of the art therapist's ongoing development.

SPACE: THE ART THERAPY ROOM

More often than not, art therapists work in less than ideal spaces. Few have the luxury of designing an art therapy room to their specifications. Although the art therapy room need not be luxurious or ideally designed, there are a few minimum requirements without which the work will suffer. These include privacy, adequate lighting and space, and freedom to mess. Many rooms of sufficient size, originally designed for other purposes, can be adapted to suit these requirements. Therefore, an art therapist should be reluctant to accept a thoroughfare, a corner of a dayroom or dining room, or some other space where she cannot meet with her patients in private. It is obvious that comings and goings of others would be intrusive or distracting, to say nothing of the difficulty in building trust when others can overhear discussion and peer at the art.

An unfortunate choice also is a room that must be used for other purposes so that patients would have to be careful not to drip paint on the carpet or get pastel dust on the upholstered furniture. Although drop cloths can be used, they tend to be cumbersome and to reinforce the need to keep the room clean. The art therapist hopes to encourage freedom of expressions rather than inhibitions around mess. The nature of art materials is that they drip, smear, get on one's hands and clothes, so it is better to prepare the environment to receive them rather than to try to keep them contained. Obviously, washable surfaces are highly desirable.

The question of room size has variable answers. If the art therapist sees only individual patients, she does not need much room. When I moved from a small office in NIH to a tiny one, one of my patients commented that she liked it better because it was cozy. It contained my desk and chair, an easel, chair for the patient, and a bookcase. There was room for nothing more. When I saw groups or families, I had to use other spaces.

A group room is best if there is adequate space for each individual to work separately without being unduly influenced by the others. I often suggest to group members that they position themselves so that they can turn away from the others to explore themselves most fully without seeing their neighbor's art expressions until all are completed. This way they are more likely to follow their own lights rather than to copy one another.

In addition to adequate space for art-making there should be the possibility for the group to join together to share and discuss the artwork. The same space used for making art usually suffices, sometimes with a rearrangement of furniture. Sessions for individual patients, of course, require little space for the art therapist and client to look at the artwork together.

Furnishings make a difference—whether art therapy participants work at easels, tables, or on the floor, whether seating is on chairs or carpet and cushions. Art therapists should sit with their patients on chairs or floor, at the same level, not above or below. Usually, the floor is conducive to a more informal atmosphere and greater relaxation. Chairs keep people more separate and apart than a common floor on which they are seated or may lounge. These are considerations for art therapists to take into account in setting up the work space.

It is desirable for the art room to contain shelves or cabinets for supplies and storage of art products, but this is not essential. If necessary, they can be transported from a nearby storage area. Also desirable is a sink for clean-up, but water, too, can be brought in.

Storage of the art products is best if there is a place for each patient's work, a folder for pictures, a shelf for sculpture. This sort of treatment of the art underscores its importance, specialness, and personal worth. The manner in which the art therapist physically handles the artwork and fashions the environment to receive it says much about the significance she gives the product and its maker. It is not likely that a patient would believe that the art therapist took art therapy seriously if she treated the artwork carelessly. Or the patient might feel she devalued him or his artwork. Out-patients and private practice clients may be asked to take their artwork with them when sufficient storage space is not available.

MATERIALS

Since this is a book about art psychotherapy rather than art-making per se, I will not attempt a discussion of all the properties of art materials. The American Art Therapy Association Guidelines for Education and Training specifies that a prerequisite for Master's Degree training in art therapy is studio art. Therefore, prior to art therapy practice, the art therapist has gained a familiarity with materials and methods. She knows surfaces, such as different papers, canvas, board; drawing materials, such as pencils, pens, charcoal, markers; color media, such as paints, pastels, craypas; three dimensional media, such as clay, plaster, wood; tools, such as paint brushes, sculpting utensils, glues. She also knows methods, such as how to keep a clay piece damp until next session or what thinner to use to make a wash from oil pastels. (Those who have specialized in only one or two areas of art-making can readily learn the necessary technical information about the other basic media and methods.)

With this sort of knowledge at her fingertips, the art therapist can then select media wisely for her clients. Knowledge of specific materials is helpful. For example, water pastels offer the advantage of using water for a thinner, but their colors are less vivid than oil pastels which require turpentine. Some materials are inherently frustrating, like newsprint which tears easily under pressure from drawing materials. Some chalks crumble easily. Clay that is not well prepared may be hard and resistant. Brushes that are old and worn make painting more difficult to control. It is obvious that materials need to be in good condition, and the art therapist can certainly urge her clients to help in cleaning up and not abusing the equipment.

In ordering materials, the art therapist makes selections based on her knowledge of the medium's properties, the needs of her clients, and the conditions under which she works. It's likely that she will want to have some variety, including drawing materials, paints, and a three-dimensional medium. For basics, I would select pastels, a water paint with properties of both poster paint and watercolors, and clay. All three can be used quickly and spontaneously without much preparation and clean-up. I generally avoid pencils because they tend to suggest writing and reinforce rigidity and constriction, as opposed to the more flowing or smearable media, such as paints and pastels.

Materials for collage provide a good addition for those who are threatened by creating. Assembling images may be easier while still personal and expressive. Combined cut-outs from magazines can tell revealing stories. All that is needed are poster paper, magazines, scissors, and Elmer's glue. For more original collage, use colored tissue paper and cellophane and watered down Elmer's glue. The overlapping of colors can produce lovely effects and help people to feel quite creative.

I give patients large paper, 18″ x 24″, because I want to encourage their expansiveness rather than constriction. The paper can always be cut to a smaller size if clients are intimidated by the larger expanse or if there is a particular reason they would like to work small. In my experience, patients have seldom changed the size, though often they have not filled the whole paper. The empty space may be an important aspect of the picture's expression, as in Figure 13.

Media and methods used in art therapy are generally simple and easy for several reasons. Usually the art therapist hopes to encourage a spontaneous release of feeling. Unconscious material is more likely to emerge if one does not have to engage in elaborate preparation or planning in tackling the media. Other factors are costs and space. For example, it is not likely that an art therapist will have equipment or room for lithography, welding, or metal casting. As is obvious from these examples, safety is a factor as well. There are advantages to media that enable completion within one session. While the feelings are still current the client can reflect on the artwork and discuss it with the art therapist. The client can leave the session with a sense of realization from expression and exploration. In a short-term treatment setting, there may not be time for continuous work on one project. Finally, an additional advantage of a simple medium is that it can be given to a client to use between sessions. A box of craypas or pastels and some paper can be easily carried to a patient's room or home, for example.

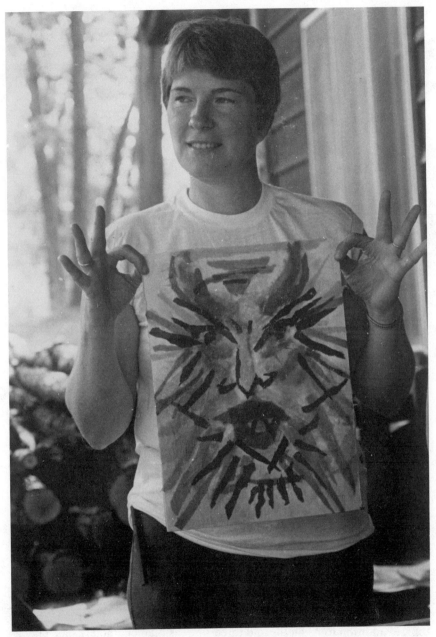

Figure 12. Tissue paper collage: Elizabeth Slenker shows her "devil."

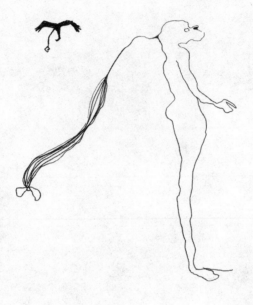

Figure 13. The importance of empty space.

Media Characteristics

In meeting patients' individual needs, there are a few salient features of particular materials and expressive dimensions that are worth underscoring for art therapy purposes. An important media characteristic is control. Some materials are easy to control, especially those that are more precise, such as pencils. In contrast, water paints offer fluidity but are difficult to control. Their sometimes accidental wanderings across the paper may offer welcome surprises for an adventurous patient or frustration for the patient who wants to maintain control of his art expression.

Commitment is another significant dimension. Some materials are indelible, such as markers. There is little possibility of undoing. At the opposite extreme is clay. It offers opportunity for endless change. Therefore, in addition to its tactile and three-dimensional characteristics, clay is an excellent medium for creating transformations.

Color intensity is a variable of media art therapists should consider. Some materials are inherently pale, such as colored pencils or water pastels, and others inherently vivid, such as markers. Therefore, in offering these media the art therapist must be aware that she is limiting her client to one or the other possibility for color intensity. Obviously, there are many other materials that facilitate more variety of expression in this regard.

Drawing or coloring is another significant factor in selecting art materials. Some media lend themselves readily to the former, such as pencils and pen and ink, and others to the latter, such as watercolors. Coloring with pencil or pen can be tedious, and drawing with water paint can be frustrating. Some media allow for both possibilities, such as craypas and pastels. An art therapist may wish to suggest a change in medium if a patient is having trouble drawing or coloring with materials unsuited to his purpose.

Gravity exerts an influence on building three-dimensional projects. A clay piece that collapses is frustrating, and ways to provide support may be needed. Technical assistance is sometimes necessary for such projects.

Large motor activity is possible in pounding clay or in hammering or sawing wood for built products. Such activity can be useful in venting strong feelings, especially anger, or in working off excess energy.

A Selection of Media

I would consider an art therapy program to be well supplied if it furnished the following:

- Pastels (I prefer AlphaColors and Grumbacher for their vivid colors, stick size, and consistency—soft enough to smear and hard enough to draw.)
- Craypas
- Markers
- Water paints and brushes (both flat and tapered)
- Clay, a few tools, boards to hold the sculpture, and plastic covering
- Paris Craft (plaster infused gauze)
- Magazines and tissue paper for collage, scissors, poster paper, and glue
- Acryllic paints, brushes, paletts, canvas, (for long term work only)

- Pastel or charcoal paper, 18″ x 24″
- Colored paper, 18″ x 24″
- Watercolor paper, 18″ x 24″

All these materials are not necessary, however. In facilities with limited budgets, excellent work can be done with just a few simple supplies such as pastels, water paint, paper, and clay. There have been situations where I have been limited to pastels and paper only (such as when I have had to hold art therapy in a patient's room or the seclusion room), yet managed to conduct very effective art therapy. Materials need to be adequate, not elaborate. The quality of the therapeutic relationship is far more important than the quality of the art supplies. It is important to keep this balance in perspective while considering media. Nevertheless, gross inadequacies in supplies can hamper the art therapy process.

Patient Needs

Properties of art materials compose the foundation knowledge necessary for any art teacher. Important in art therapy is the matching of this knowledge with sensitivity to the patient's condition and needs. Timing is often a factor. For example, there may be occasions when one would want to bolster defenses and support a choice by the patient of a more rigid or constrictive medium. At another time, one might wish to encourage the same patient to break through some of the defenses, to be less controlled, to try something different with a less easily controlled medium. In most instances, I leave the choice of medium to the client, but there might be occasions when I would suggest using a different medium. If a person is particularly frustrated with one medium, I might offer another, or help the patient confront the difficulty in the original medium. A more frequent cause for me to suggest a change is when an individual appears in a rut, perhaps making the same stereotyped image over and over again. But even this occasion is relatively rare. Some people like to experiment in trying various media. Others establish a comfort with one and stick with it, finding it a useful vehicle for the development of their images. I seldom interfere with these selections.

Choice of medium is likely to be more crucial for children than for adults. Children are more prone to dive in without regard for their own limitations, time constraints, and so forth. Therefore, they may need assistance in planning feasible use of media. Particularly at issue is whether one might wish to encourage regression or not, by use of such materials as finger paints or squishy clay. Adults who are invested in an

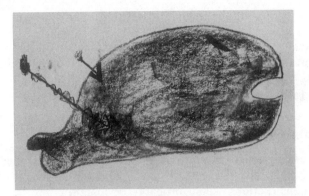

Figure 14. Technical assistance helped a six-year-old boy to open his whale's mouth.

art project seldom fly to pieces if the project does not work out, whereas children sometimes do. In my experience, adults have torn up a picture or smashed a sculpture when its contents has been distressing to them, rather than when frustrated with their inability to make what they wanted.

Technical Assistance

Frustration in creating art raises the question of instruction or guidance. Since the goal is not artistic accomplishment, but rather self-expression, there is no place in art therapy for art instruction. An art therapist would certainly give a mixed message if she criticized an art object for elements of composition. On the other hand, there may be moments when technical assistance is required. A child with whom I was working was having difficulty with runny paints at the easel. I showed him how to catch the drips with an almost dry brush. Another child had made a mark with pastel he wanted to erase. It only smeared. I showed him how to go over it with white (Figure 14, the whale's mouth that had originally been drawn closed).

Since the artwork is self-expression, the art therapist neither makes suggestions for its development nor works on it herself.* Even if the client asks for such assistance, she should respond by indicating that it is the client's picture or sculpture and help the client to decide the choice in question. For example, if the client is drawing his family and asks if he should include his aunt, the art therapist might ask how he feels about his aunt, does he consider her a part of the family, and so forth. If he asks

* Exceptions are discussed in Chapter 5.

how to draw a horse, she might suggest that he try to visualize what a horse looks like.

Additionally, it is probably not even necessary to add that with a goal of self-expression, the art therapist does not offer preplanned projects like painting-by-the-numbers or molds into which clay can be poured or patterns for craft projects such as leather belts and wallets.

Context of Art Therapy

The art therapist must take into account the conditions of her work regarding art materials. If she works on a short-term unit, oil painting or elaborate constructions would probably be inappropriate because there would not be time for completing the project. If she is working with a relatively large group or with disruptive patients, she had best keep materials simple. If a treatment goal is socialization, she might try group mural work. If she is working in a facility for the physically impaired, she must be sensitive to her clients' physical limitations and use materials that her clients can handle, sometimes modifying their usual method of application. For example, Cherie Natenberg, a student working with a partially paralyzed woman, designed an innovative Velcro® strap to help her hold a paint brush, Figure 15. Work with this woman is described further in Chapter 9.

Media Projects

Although simple basic media stock a program that can suit most art therapy services, it is also possible for art therapists to engage clients in innovative projects. These activities can range from a simple use of materials to complex projects. As always, the art therapist selects activities purposefully with the needs and abilities of her clients in mind as well as the resources the setting offers. Many of the materials that can be used are inexpensive and easily available. They include: magazines and tissue paper for collage; cardboard for constructions that can be painted; newspaper and starch or paste for papier maché that can be molded and painted; scrap wood for construction that can be painted; Paris Craft plaster infused gauze for molding that can be painted and decorated with other materials; plaster for construction; fabric for puppets, costumes, and other objects; pipe cleaners for construction; polaroid photographs that can be included as a part of other artwork. Where the project is relatively complex and time-consuming, art therapy is geared toward the art-making process, often with more investment in creating a product than is involved in quick spontaneous picture-making.

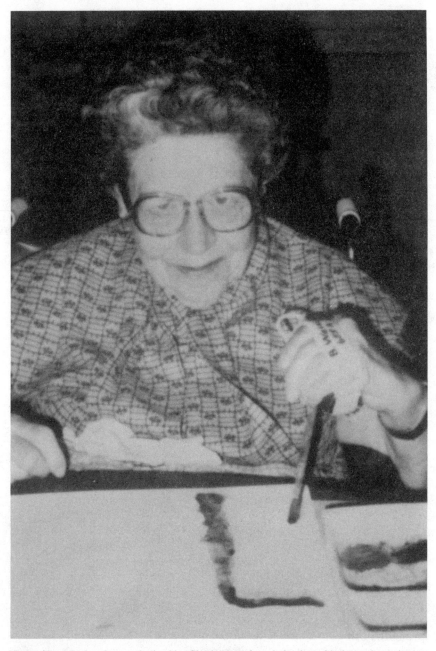

Figure 15. A Velcro® strap devised by Cherie Natenberg helped an elderly stroke patient to hold a paint brush.

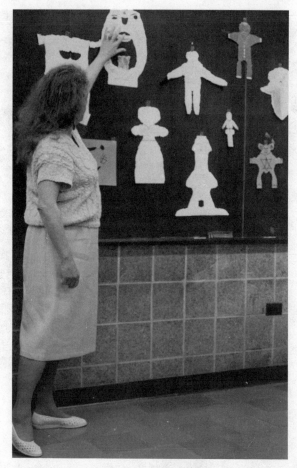

Figure 16. Prisoners' self-portraits.

The possibilities for innovative use of materials in art therapy projects is extensive. In order to illustrate a range of activities from simple to complex, a few examples are presented here. The first is very simple and demonstrates what can be done when a needed tool is prohibited. Nancy Hadley worked with jail inmates who were not allowed scissors. In order to provide a group of these men a self-expressive experience, she suggested that they fold paper in half and tear out self-portraits, Figure 16. After unfolding them, some made additional tears. This simple activity promoted self-expression without the necessity for artistic skill or experience, or even the customary cutting tool.

There are times when the art therapist may wish the client to have a satisfying experience and a feeling of mastery in creating a product of which he can be proud. Such may be the case in working with a child who is readily discouraged with his own efforts. Some materials are easily worked and often produce good results even though their creators' abilities, concentration, or patience may be limited. I'm not referring to prepared molds or numbered paintings, but rather personal self-expressive products. Magazine and tissue paper collages are of this nature, as described previously.

Gauze-infused plaster (Paris Craft) is also a material that can be used successfully. A more complex and extensive project than collage-making, Paris Craft molds of objects from life offer interesting possibilities. One of them is mask-making. Masks provide opportunity for projecting, confronting, and exploring aspects of the self. In using Paris Craft, work with the self is highlighted through molding the mask from one's own face. Such an activity can promote intimate pairing as well, as one applies the wet gauze plaster to the face of another, as shown in Figure 17. An additional advantage is the opportunity to transform a self-representation with additional plaster, paint, or decorative objects (Figures 1, 9).

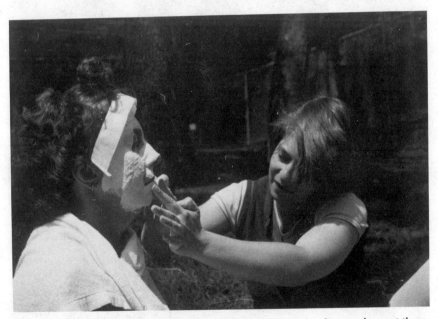

Figure 17. Student Deborah Neilsen forms a paris-craft plaster bandage mask on art therapist Kay Cox's face.

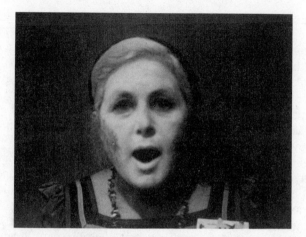

Figure 18. The author in clown white face.

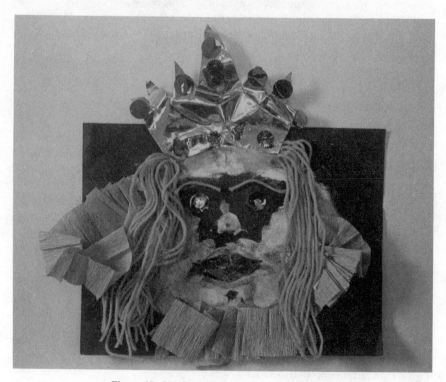

Figure 19. Mask made from print of white face.

Another mask project that utilizes simple materials is one developed by Elizabeth Spear Rogers for work with children. First one applies clown white grease paint to the face, Figure 18. Polaroid pictures of this step enhance the connection between one's actual face and the mask. Then black paper is pressed against the face to make a print. Next the print is decorated. Figure 19 is my experience with this process. I wrote the following about this self-image:

Her Highness Harriet

This is me trying to be something or someone I'm not. I appear over-done, ridiculous, and sort of pathetic.

Mask-making can lead to self-expressive dramatic play, a particularly important activity for children. Other such possibilities include puppets that promote first the making of a self-expressive project, and then the opportunity to utilize it in enactment. Figure 20 shows art therapist Ellen Sontag demonstrating covering a balloon with plaster gauze to form the head to which material is then added for the body that covers the puppet-eers hand, Figure 21. Expressive puppet faces can also be made from stuffed nylon stockings, Figure 22. Scraps of varied materials offer many possibilities for costuming the puppets.

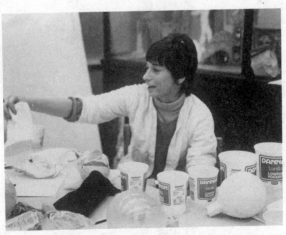

Figure 20. Ellen Sontag demonstrates puppet-making.

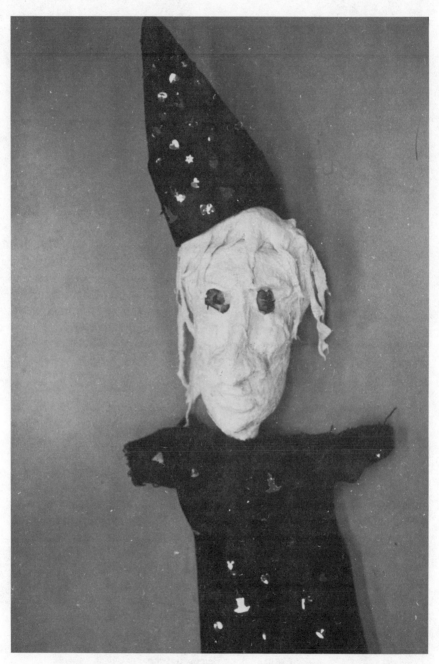

Figure 21. Puppet made from plaster gauze-covered balloon.

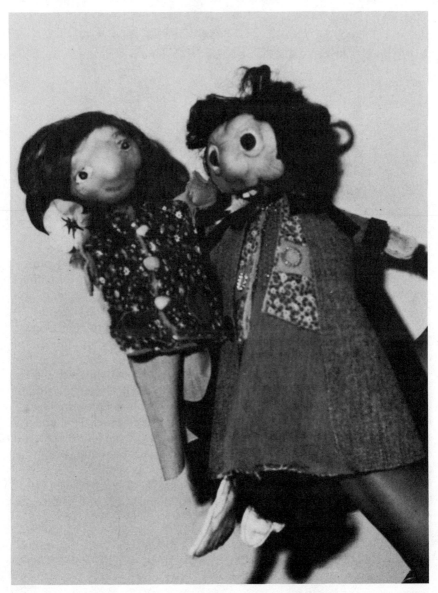

Figure 22. Stocking face puppets are individual expressions that can be used for enactment as well.

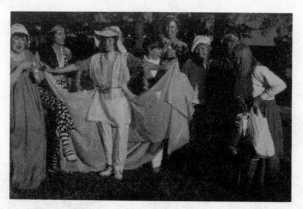

Figure 23. Creative costuming can be expressive.

Use of fabrics suggests many innovative projects. Costuming can include the self, as well as puppets, and leads to creative transformations that even adults can enjoy, as seen in Figure 23. In puppet play, one becomes the puppet, giving it a voice and action. On the other hand, fabric can also be used to create a doll with which one can interact. Figure 24 shows a sorrowful doll made by Elizabeth Day that can be spoken to, cuddled, and comforted.

An ambitious puppet/drama project is the creation of over-size puppets from heavy cardboard sometimes fortified with wood. These larger-than-life images are often used for pageants or ritual dramas rather than more intimate dramatic play. Figure 25 is an autumn ritual procession created by Chicago's Big Fish Celebration Theatre showing, from left to right, the queen, the dragon, a labyrinth, and the hero. These creations and the ritual enactment of which they were a part served as symbolic metaphors for the participants' own individual hero journeys. The final pageant followed weeks of preparation involving creating, enacting, and self-exploration.

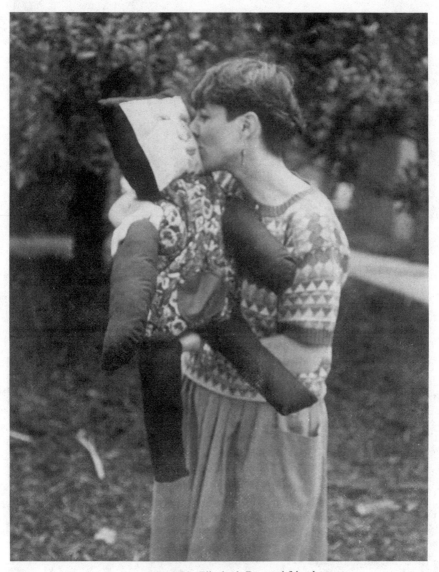

Figure 24. Elizabeth Day and friend.

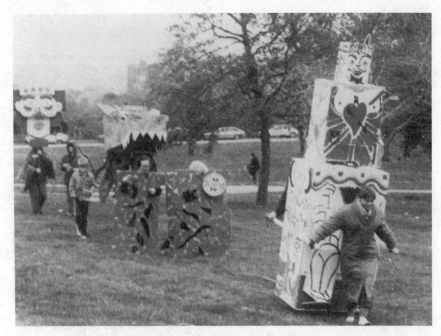

Figure 25. Oversize puppets in autumn ritual pageant.

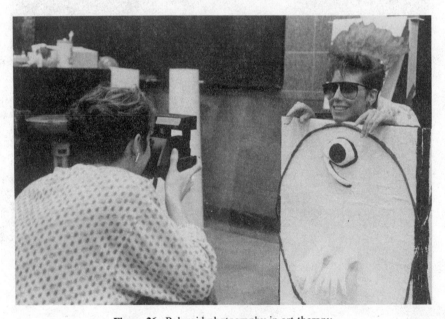

Figure 26. Polaroid photography in art therapy.

The final example of more exotic art therapy projects takes us into our high-tech age. Polaroid photography, though necessitating expensive equipment, provides a fascinating self-reference. Requiring no technical ability, the picture-making process itself offers unique opportunities for pairing and creating a setting, Figure 26. Either the photographer or the person photographed can compose and direct the shot. The photograph can then be embellished in a larger image, Figure 27. An object in the photograph can be cut out before mounting, and multiple images can be used as well. The power of photography used in this way is its unique self-referent quality. Equally compelling is the opportunity it provides the individual to select and arrange meaningful objects in the environment. Claudia Clenard, photographing in Figure 26, used the polaroid camera

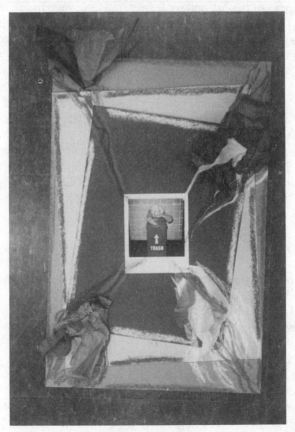

Figure 27. Polaroid portrait, embellished in mounting.

extensively in art therapy with psychiatrically hospitalized adolescents. Being put in restraints was an impactful experience for many of them, and they used the camera in simulating this event. The creations that evolved from these images were important landmarks in helping these patients to process the experience of their illness.

In sum, the art therapist combines her knowledge of art materials with her sensitivity to her clients' conditions and needs during any particular session within the framework of the conditions under which she works to select suitable materials most facilitating to the art therapy process for each individual client.

Art Materials and Transference

A subtle aspect of the art materials picture is its place in the transference relationship (discussed at greater length in Chapter 5). The art therapist comes to be seen as the provider of supplies. One adolescent patient I saw at the NIH entered the art therapy room for the first time as though she were arriving in heaven. She had been making art for many years and could hardly believe that all the materials I had would be at her disposal "for free." At that moment, I was the beneficent mother to her, giving her more than she could possible use. On the other hand, one of my students introduced art therapy to a facility that did not come up with sufficient funds for art supplies. She was given some meager leftover broken crayons and small, poor quality paper. As a result of this and other nonsupportive conditions, her patients came to experience her as a more withholding parent. (Since this facility did not live up to its agreements with our training program, it was soon terminated as a placement site for our students.)

When I saw groups in private practice, I asked participants to bring their own art materials, rather than to supply them as is the case in institutional settings. There were several reasons for this. One was that I wanted to keep the fee as low as possible, and by not providing art materials, I did not have to add that expense to the fee. But more significant was the message I wished to give. These group members were well-functioning professionals, some of them artists and art therapists. I wanted to encourage them to be responsible for their equipment needs rather than to encourage dependency. On the other hand, the reaction of the adolescent previously described evidenced the sort of nourishment a protective environment can give to those who are too dependent to live outside the hospital at the time. The method of supplying the art materials, therefore, can serve to encourage the nature of the transference relationship.

In most instances, then, the art therapist gives not only of her attention, interest, understanding, and care, as other therapists do, but also tangible material supplies. Further, they are given unconditionally—patients can do with them as they wish (aside from using them abusively or destructively, of course).

A hospitalized adolescent decided he wanted to throw oil paint and clay against the wall. We covered it with brown paper. He fashioned hollow clay pellets about three inches long with a hole in the end. When they were dry, he squirted a different color oil paint in each. In an explosive burst of pleasure he threw them vehemently one by one against the wall. He was able to release feeling, make "a big splash," and be destructive without doing any damage. I was able to assist him in his project rather than hold him back because of an unorthodox use of the materials. This example illustrates the way in which an art therapist can facilitate expression and freedom rather than being a watchdog over "proper" use of materials. In regard to transference, she may all too readily fit the preexperienced mold of the strict, inhibiting teacher.

The art therapist needs to be sensitive to the place her responsibility for art supplies may hold in the transference relationship with individual clients. The materials may be experienced as extensions of the art therapist and treated accordingly, tentatively with great care and fear, with relish and indulgence, taken for granted, disregarded, or abused. Although I have worked with close to 100 nonmedicated acute schizophrenics and full-blown manics, I have never had an art therapy session where the patient was so destructive of the materials that we had to stop. Sometimes boundaries are tested, however, such as by the patient who "accidentally" kept spilling the paint. In most instances where there is negative transference acted out on the art materials, there is also a mixture of positive response to being given to. It would be a mistake, however, to assume that the materials always stand for the art therapist. Sometimes they are treated as the institution's equipment and are related to accordingly or simply as art supplies independent of transference phenomena. This is one of many questions necessitating the art therapist's sensitivity.

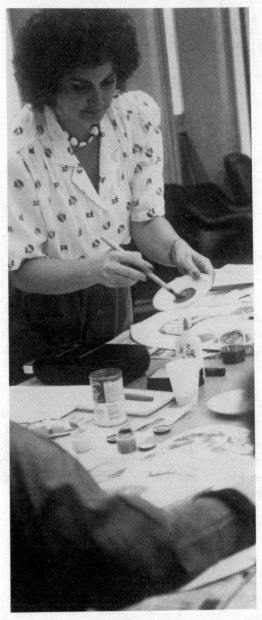

Figure 28. Cherie Natenberg mixes paint for her elderly clients.

CHAPTER 3

Encouraging Art Expression

CREATING THE CREATIVE/THERAPEUTIC ENVIRONMENT/ENCOUNTER

Creativity comes naturally to all of us. If you observe young children, you can see them interact with their environment first by exploring—looking, touching, tasting—then by manipulating objects. Initially, the motions might be relatively random. Later, they become purposeful. With increasing age comes inventiveness—games, stories, pictures, increasingly intricate forms of play. This potentiality for the shaping of experience and fantasy does not die with the loss of childhood. But it may become funneled into channels of socialization. A natural growth toward mastery (such as the child's inevitable struggle to walk) may be transformed from a desired end in itself to the service of approved accomplishment. For example, what might be a young person's physical pleasure in exercising, developing strength and coordination, may be channeled into an effort to "make the team."

In making art, young children start by playing with the materials and may be hardly interested in the product. With advancing age, this exploration becomes manipulation, and eventually purposeful inventiveness in the fashioning of a product. The feelings of pride, power, and control for the previously helpless infant provide a compelling incentive to create.

Art production is a special sort of creativity. One makes a product, creates a world or a piece of world. The creator can stand back and admire the creation. There is an interesting paradox here. The creation is an expression of self, an extension of self. And yet the creator can be separate from that aspect of self, can look at it, touch it, move it, even walk away from it and come back later, or never see it again. It is both a part of self and separate. It has been created by one's own mastery, out of one's own uniqueness. There is a sense of personal power here—"I did that!" Have you ever seen a child's face upon the completion of such a work? Have you ever seen that "I did that!" look of pride? Often such a reaction follows a process that is very absorbing. Many times when I am engrossed in art, the world melts away. Preoccupations dissolve in the intensity of my focus. Usually when I stop I am surprised at how much time has passed.

The point I am trying to make is that the process art therapists encourage is a natural one. If there had not been interference in our lives, there would probably be no need for art therapists. Since there has been interference, often the task of the art therapist is to help remove the roadblocks to the natural flow of creativity.

REMOVING ROADBLOCKS

Performance Fear

One of the greatest roadblocks to creative self-expression is performance fear. This is an expectable anxiety in our product/achievement-oriented society. For example, I approached my Ph.D. project (the equivalent of a dissertation) with heavy foreboding. It was going to be hard *work*. My faculty advisor, Roy Fairfield, said to me: "Muck around for a while." That was the most liberating statement anyone could have made to me. The burden of *work* was lifted from me and I could now *play* with my project. What I was attempting to do was to integrate many years of art therapy practice into a book. That book had been sitting on my shoulders (and they actually ached!) for several years. But I simply could not begin. In an effort to confront my resistance, I wrote a dialogue in letters between my book and myself. What I learned in the course of this dialogue was that I wanted my book to be the definitive statement of Harriet Wadeson, the professional. No wonder I was paralyzed! But my book was kind to me. It told me to enjoy myself, to write to please no one but myself, to put it aside if I got bored with it, and to discard it completely if I didn't enjoy it. The result of this invitation to play and the release from the oppression of trying to write a book representing the perfect art therapy professional resulted in a completed first draft within three months! The contents of *Art Psychotherapy* (1980) had taken form within me over the years. All that was needed was to unlock the barriers to allow my ideas to come flowing out of my head, down my arm, through my pen onto the paper.

The same sort of process can happen in the art therapy session. I often invite patients to play, to experiment with the media, not to worry about

making a picture. They explore possibilities rather than produce something. Together we explore meaning rather than produce meaning. It's
okay if we don't find meaning. After all, it was only an experiment. Often
there's a shared excitement as art therapist and client venture together
into this world of surprises. Because an approach of playfulness usually
brings with it a freeing up of spontaneity, we are likely to be greeted by
the unexpected, by the more meaningful. This is one of the paradoxes in
art therapy. Trying to produce a meaningful product can impede its development. Relaxing into play more likely encourages the emergence of what
is within to flow out into art expression.

It goes without saying that the art therapist's meta-message to the
patient is one of acceptance rather than judgment. The fear of judgment,
of course, is at the base of performance anxiety. So the meta-message
would be "I'm interested in your picture" rather than "This picture is
better than last week's." The communication of the desired meta-message is seldom achieved with one statement alone, but is built up over
experience so that the patient comes to understand any one comment in a
context of the art therapist's consistent approach to the patient and the
art. If the meta-message is to be interest rather than judgment, the art
therapist is well advised to avoid positive comments as well as criticisms
about artistic merit. Although such a practice might appear withholding,
many individuals seek approval and when it is given sometimes and not
others they may assume an implied criticism when approval is absent.
The meta-message, once again, is more appropriately interest in the patient's experience rather than in artistic accomplishment. Praise, therefore, is more beneficially given for hard therapeutic work or therapeutic
progress, because that is the goal. The goal of artistic accomplishment
belongs to the art class rather than to art therapy.

Mr. Gump, an elderly patient hospitalized at the National Institutes of
Health Clinical Center for agitated depression, provides a dramatic example of performance fear and experimentation. Mr. Gump had been a
draftsman but in his depressed state was convinced he had lost all ability
to do anything, including drawing. At our first session he paced the room
without stopping, muttered incomprehensibly, and refused to look at either the art materials or me. At the second session, he was less agitated,
but refused to touch the art media, repeating that he could no longer draw.
I encouraged him to see what the charcoal and pastels would feel like—
not to draw a picture. He told me about the famous art school he had
attended 50 years ago. As we spoke about it he picked up a piece of
charcoal and made some marks on a corner of the stack of drawing paper,
still not approaching the paper affixed to the easel for him. At the next

Figure 29. "Nonpicture" by a resistant depressed man, Mr. Gump.

session he continued to reminisce about art school and on the bottom of a piece of paper in the supply stack he demonstrated the way he had been taught to draw a head, Figure 29. He was not making a picture. He was just showing me something. At the next session he spoke about the land-scapes he had liked to draw when he used to be able to do so. He demon-strated with charcoal on a corner of the supply stack paper. Next he approached the easel and started one in charcoal, Figure 30. Shortly thereafter he began to fill the paper as he drew with sustained attention, Figure 31. A couple of sessions later, he tried color. He became less agitated on the ward. He was eager for art therapy sessions. He asked his wife to bring in some of the paintings he had made in the past. He began doing artwork outside the sessions.

Throughout Mr. Gump's life his art expression had been realistic, de-tailed, meticulous, with little personal expression. Nevertheless, instead of sticking with what was familiar, successful, and easily controlled, he began to experiment. He built an easel in occupational therapy and made a colorful abstract picture intricately executed in pastels to be exhibited on it, Figure 32. He made a "death mask" in clay. He drew a smoldering volcano and reflected that it was himself, Figure 33. His psychiatrist said to me, "Harriet, you've cured Mr. Gump." More accurately, I furnished the encouragement and environment for Mr. Gump to "cure" himself.

It's interesting to note that in this instance there was very little attempt to utilize insight in treatment. A depleted man rediscovered strengths. An isolated individual found he could connect with others. Therapy occurred through his doing more than through his understanding. Mr. Gump over-

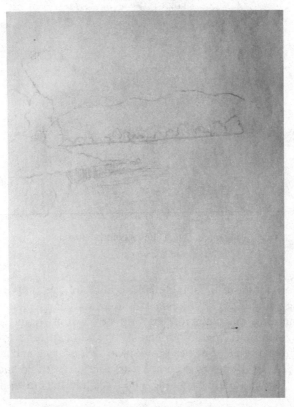

Figure 30. Tentative landscape by Mr. Gump.

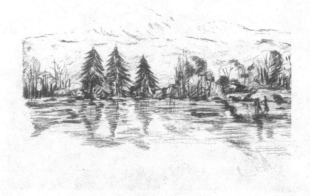

Figure 31. Mr. Gump's black and white landscape.

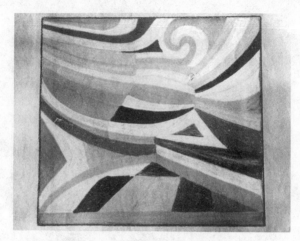

Figure 32. Mr. Gump's colorful abstract.

came his conviction of incompetence because he was only explaining or showing me something, not feeling pressured to make a picture. This sort of experimenting environment led him beyond previous abilities. He found enjoyment in trying out unfamiliar ways to express himself as well.

Mr. Gump was a person with previous art experience and ability. What about most of the others who come to art therapy with no such art backgrounds? In my experience, people who have had the most anxiety about

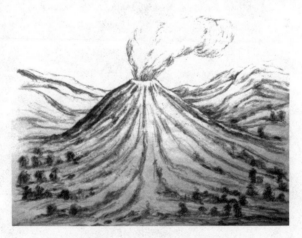

Figure 33. Volcano by Mr. Gump.

their performance have been patients hospitalized for psychotic depression. Most have felt worthless and hopeless. They have assumed that their art would show their inability, childishness, and would be meaningless. Often as well, they have been physically lethargic and apathetic. Nevertheless, having worked with over 100 psychotically depressed patients, I have never had a patient who refused altogether to try art expression, though some, such as Mr. Gump, did not do so in the first session. The following statement made by a suicidal woman who had no art ability sums up her experience: "At first I thought art therapy was silly and childish, but I really got a lot out of making these pictures even though I never did learn how to draw."

Fear of Self-Revelation

Fear of self-revelation may be another roadblock. Often, there are fantasies that the art therapist can "read" the art. In response, the art therapist demonstrates that the patient does most of the interpreting. Understanding the art is a collaborative venture in which art therapist and patient explore together the possibilities of meaning. In time the patient comes to see that the art therapist is not going to make assumptions from the art. Even when art therapy is not insight-oriented, the therapist can comment on the art to let the patient know her response, thereby helping to dispel some of his fantasies about her reactions. For example, she might say, "This picture looks as though more is happening in it than the one you did last week. Is that your impression, too?" The patient may then go on to discuss it further or not, depending on his readiness to do so.

Who Sees the Art

A part of the fear of self-revelation may be concern over who else will see the art. At the outset, the art therapist should make clear (even if the patient doesn't ask) who will see the art productions and under what circumstances. Will they be brought to staff meetings? Will they be shown to the patient's psychiatrist? Will they ever be shown to family members? Obviously, feelings of trust are more likely to develop in an atmosphere of openness rather than secrecy about who sees the art.

Decisions about showing the artwork are influenced by many factors. In a setting utilizing a team approach, it would be deleterious for the art therapist not to share information with the other team members. On the other hand, showing artwork to family members might diminish the possibility of building a therapeutic alliance based on trust. This would be particularly true in the case of adolescent patients. In work with very young children, however, it might be beneficial to parents in understanding their children to see their artwork and to hear the art therapist's comments about the child's needs. Nevertheless, a child's "secrets" should be respected. Young children, of course, have less concern about judgment of their spontaneous self-expression than do more socialized older children and adults, who themselves have become more product- and achievement-oriented. In most cases, the art expression is usually considered confidential communication and treated accordingly.

Art Displays

Many art therapists display patient artwork both to give the patient a sense of pride and accomplishment and to encourage further art expression. Decisions in this area need to be considered carefully. I tend not to display patient art. The meta-message I am trying to convey is that the art expression in art therapy is experimental, not product-oriented, and is a personal self-expression and communication. If patients wish to show their artwork, they are free to do so. Some who were hospitalized took their art to other staff, patients, and family. Some gave their work away as gifts. The choice was theirs. There was never even an implicit expectation that they "produce" an object of artistic merit. Most of the people with whom I have worked, including some artists, have used art therapy as a personal journey inwards facilitated by and shared with an art therapist.

Lack of Choice

Another significant resistance is in the anger a patient may feel in being forced into an unwanted situation. This may be the result of being required to participate in art therapy or being coerced into treatment as a whole. In either case, art therapy is a fine place to offer resistance. After all, a person cannot be forced to produce art in the same way a patient may be force-fed medication or locked on a hospital ward. Those who are more passive-aggressive may comply with the request to draw but execute something so minimal that the message of defiance is all too clear.

So what does the art therapist do? As always, she tries to build a therapeutic alliance. The worst thing she can do is engage in a power struggle. She can let the patient know that she understands the feelings of anger about being coerced to do what you don't want to do. She might encourage a ventilation of these feelings. At first this may be done in the more comfortable verbal mode. The patient may be angry at particular people. The art therapist can show her interest in understanding the patient's predicament. Eventually she may encourage the patient to express some of these feelings through the art media. The point here is the building of an alliance rather than an opposition. That is the prime consideration—not whether the patient engages in art or not. It may take several sessions until the patient trusts that this activity might be beneficial, or at minimum, that he is not being forced to participate.

POSITIVE INCENTIVES

This section has concentrated on roadblocks, because they are most apparent; and often it is only their removal that is necessary to encourage positive participation in art therapy. But there are many inducements as well. Most of them are obvious.

SPACE.   An inviting space with adequate lighting, enough room to work, but not so vast as to feel empty, suitable equipment easily cleaned up, quiet, and privacy facilitate art expression and communication. A room that is poorly lit, noisy, too cramped, lacking in necessary equipment, clearly interferes with ease in engagement in art therapy. Logistical considerations can make an enormous difference. Often art therapists are not so fortunate as to be able to work under ideal conditions and must utilize their creativity in arranging the space they do have. (Specific considerations are discussed in Chapter 2.)

ART MATERIALS.   The particular properties and potentialities of various media are discussed in Chapter 2. To encourage art expression they should be in good condition and readily accessible. If they are difficult to find or jumbled together with other supplies, they may not be used. For example, a patient with low energy who has decided to use poster paint may give up after being unable to locate a brush and discovering the paints to be all dried out. For some patients supplies may need to be arranged invitingly. Too many choices might overwhelm some. The art therapist must be sensitive to these factors and present the art materials accordingly.

Art Therapeutic Relationship

By far the most important factor, however, is the way in which the art therapist relates to the client or patient to encourage art expression. Many art therapists have had to work in inadequate space with meager art supplies and yet managed to do very effective work.

I usually introduce patients to art therapy by telling them that it provides another way to express yourself in addition to words. I say that I don't expect them to have any particular art experience or talent. I might then say something about the art materials I have set out. Usually, I begin with pastels because they are quick, easy, versatile, and have inviting vivid colors. Often I tell the client that the pastels can be used for both coloring and drawing and that one color may be used on top of another to produce new colors. Sometimes I demonstrate, but usually this introduction is sufficient. With resistant patients, however, I try to determine what roadblocks may be getting in the way and deal with them.

I believe the most important element is the art therapist's attitude. As the art therapist member of the treatment team, if you consider your *raison d'etre* to be to get the patient to make art, you may find yourself in a power struggle with a resistant individual. If, on the other hand, your goal is to establish rapport and come to have some understanding of the person with whom you are working, you will be more relaxed about the art. In working with hundreds of people over the years, I can remember only one who refused to make art altogether, and I think I saw her in only one or two sessions. On the other hand, there certainly have been sessions where patients did not make art, sometimes because they preferred to spend it talking, and sometimes because they were too uncomfortable with art-making.

In the latter instance (mentioned earlier), often it is helpful to encourage patients just to experiment with the materials rather than to make a picture. Sometimes they may need time to become familiar with the new environment of the art room and, most particularly, the new person, the art therapist. I often spend time on our just getting to know each other. If the patient is more comfortable talking, we may do quite a bit before I suggest, "Why don't you try to put that feeling (experience) into a picture."

The important elements of the art encouragement aspect of the therapeutic relationship are the meta-messages the art therapist is conveying. They should be: "I am interested in you; I want to understand you; I want to see you and your world as they appear to you." One hopes, they are never: "Because I am the art therapist and I say art-making is good for you, you should do it; I'm going to assess (evaluate, diagnose) you on the basis of your art; if patients refuse to make art, I'll be out of a job."

Frequently there is something subtly seductive in a positive way in what the art therapist is offering. In early childhood, mother may have watched us make various kinds of productions in a similarly caring way. As adults, we seldom receive this sort of loving and singularly focussed attention. If the art therapist does her best to provide a nurturing, non-threatening environment, the resistant patient usually becomes willing to take the risk of a commitment to a mark on paper.

The next step is crucial. It is important that the art therapist respond to the art-making in an encouraging way. In the first place, she doesn't interfere with its development. She doesn't hover over the patient or initiate conversation that might be distracting. Although these injunctions may seem too obvious to state, I was surprised to see a highly respected art therapist not only hover over a withdrawn child who was painting, but eventually even paint on the child's picture, unbidden.

In responding to the finished product, the art therapist conveys interest, but does not try to "nail" the patient. She may suggest some ways for the patient to understand his art expression (more about this in Chapter 5). It is useful to say something positive, understanding, or appreciative, such as: "I think it took a lot of courage to put those scary feelings in a picture." "Being hospitalized must be very difficult for you." "Thank you for sharing such personal feelings with me."

Once clients or patients have overcome the initial hurdle of tackling art expression, even if only minimally, I have never encountered problems in their continuing to do so. As art therapy becomes a familiar activity, new media and approaches may be introduced. For those people who need little guidance, their self-determination can be fostered by eventually presenting all the materials and possibilities of working to them, and encouraging them to make their own decisions about their art activities.

Now that the art-making is underway, the next question is: What does the art therapist do with it? That is the subject of the next two chapters.

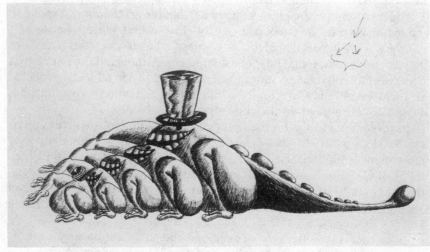

Figure 34. Whimsey in a drawing by a schizophrenic young man.

CHAPTER 4

Understanding Art Expression

What does a picture say? What does a piece of sculpture convey? In art therapy the artwork is usually viewed in a complex context that includes the client's behavior during the session, comments about the artwork, the structure of the session, the client's past history, immediate life events, relationship with the art therapist, comparisons with other artwork the client has produced, the treatment matrix in which the art therapy occurs, and so forth. (These factors are discussed in other chapters of this book.) Nevertheless, the artwork is a visual communication on its own. It's possible for an art therapist (and others as well) to look at an art expression, with no knowledge of its creator or the circumstances of its creation, and to receive a message from it.

Unfortunately, many misjudgments are made through a lack of sensitivity to the art's visual properties (sometimes accompanied by an overdependence on the client's behavior and comments) or the opposite extreme of reading into the art unfounded interpretations. Art is so rich in its expression that it is not necessary to make speculative leaps of the imagination which often produce interpretations that say more about the therapist than the clients. The full understanding of the art expression requires two skills: sensitivity to visual communication and encouragement of the client to relate to the art production. This chapter deals with the former—the visual properties of art expression in art therapy.

It is surprising that despite the diversity and sometimes controversy in understanding or interpreting patients' art, little has been written about how one may go about it. The paucity of information is especially striking when one considers the importance of this subject to art therapy practice. The reason can be found, perhaps, in the difficulty of the undertaking. Nevertheless, the following is an effort to make headway in this area.

In viewing an art expression, the art therapist receives its impact globally, not characteristic by characteristic. Sometimes particular features will be especially salient, however, such as the disorganization in Figure 35, the content of Figure 36, the empty amorphous quality of Figure 37. Each of these characteristics is the sort of visual property to which an art

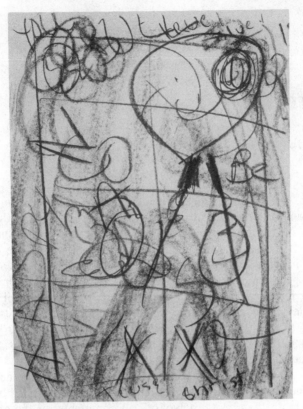

Figure 35. A schizophrenic's disorganized drawing.

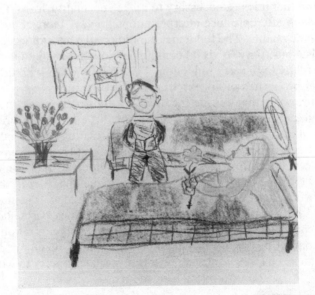

Figure 36. Explicit content in a schizophrenic young woman's drawing.

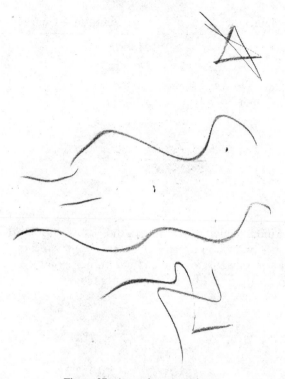

Figure 37. Amorphous emptiness.

therapist is sensitive. Although the impact of visual expression is always received in its totality, it is necessary for discussion to examine individual characteristics separately, as follows:

Pictorial Characteristics	Sculptural Characteristics
Medium	Medium
Organization	Size
Use of space, balance	Utility
Form	Construction
Color	Use of space: mass, negative space
Line	Soundness of structure, permanence
Focus or direction	Texture
Motion	Focus or direction

(*continued*)

Pictorial Characteristics	Sculptural Characteristics
Detail	Motion
Content	Detail
Affect	Content
Investment of effort	Affect
	Investment of effort

PICTORIAL CHARACTERISTICS

Medium

Obviously, choice of media determines the nature of the art expression. As this is not a book about art-making per se, I will not dwell on the properties of the various art media, but rather point out some of the attributes the art therapist takes into account.

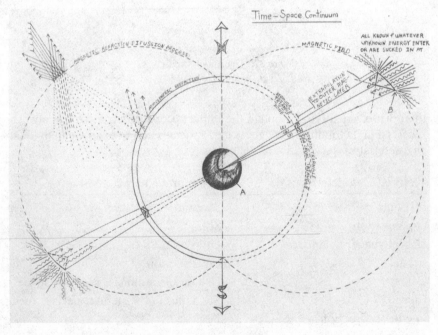

Figure 38. "Bermuda Triangle" by a schizophrenic young man.

Control

Usually, hard media are more easily controlled, such as pencils. In Figure 38 we can see that this patient left nothing to chance in a carefully thought-out scheme executed first in pencil then meticulously drawn over in ink. We need to know nothing about the patient to recognize his precise control and careful planning. Compare his picture to Figure 39 made with water paints in which we can see that the patient has allowed the paint to run. Without any additional information, we can see that this patient was spontaneous in her approach. However, she did not allow the running to get out of hand, but rather made use of its flowing quality. (Both patients were in their early 20s; both were hospitalized for acute schizophrenia; and both were delusional at the time these pictures were made.)

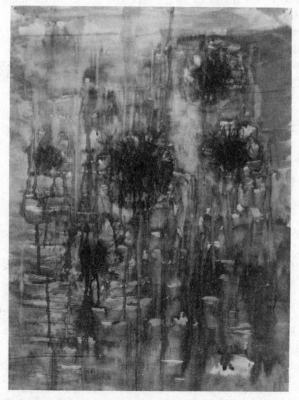

Figure 39. Lights flashing painted in water colors by a schizophrenic young woman.

Color

Some media promote use of color and others, such as pencils, ink, and charcoal, don't. In Figure 39 the patient made full use of the paint's color potential with beautiful combinations of blue and yellow. She did not allow the paint to run together so much that colors became indistinguishable or muddy. Intensity of color is also influenced by the medium used. Water pastels cannot achieve the vividness of craypas or markers, for example. Nevertheless, use of a thinner, such as water or turpentine with paints, and pressure in application of craypas or pastels for example, allow for determination of intensity.

Drawing or Coloring

Pencils, pens, and fine markers tend toward linear compositions and lend themselves to drawing, whereas water paints and large pastels are most likely used to cover areas of space (see the contrast between Figures 38 and 39 in this regard.) With pastels, colors can be smeared across the paper, whereas with craypas they cannot.

As we can see, the patients who created Figures 38 and 39, despite being hospitalized, delusional, nonmedicated acute schizophrenics at the time, were able to select appropriate media to suit their purposes and to make optimal use of the particular properties each medium provided. An art therapist sensitive to these considerations would recognize the significant strengths of these two patients, despite their bizarre behavior at the time.

Organization

A picture's organization offers information about control. Figure 38 evidences a need for tight control. One might infer a rigidity that may be a defense against fear of loss of control. Figure 35 is chaotic and indicates the patient's inability to control herself at this time. Figure 40 is neither overly controlled nor out of control. The patients who produced these pictures were all psychotic at the time. The woman who drew Figure 40 was in the midst of a manic episode, but her picture is nowhere near as disorganized as her behavior and reflects her capacity for purposeful activity, not evidenced elsewhere.

Use of Space, Balance

Is the composition arranged symmetrically giving an impression of stability and balance, as in Figure 41, despite its bizarre content? Or is it

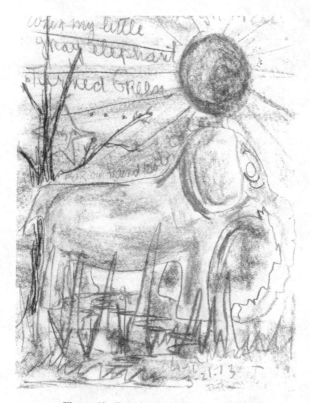

Figure 40. Drawing by a manic woman.

weighted toward the top, bottom, right, or left? Are some areas full and other parts empty? How much of the surface is covered? There seems to be a natural tendency to balance a picture so that when this is not the case, we note a lopsided effect, as in Figure 42. In this case, it appears that the people are crowded to one side of the page. We don't know if this picture was poorly planned or if there was purpose in this arrangement.

Form

Note the contrast between the formed quality of Figure 41 and the amorphousness of Figure 37. In the former we can see that the patient had a clear mental image of what he wanted to express and the ability to execute it. In the latter we see some attempt at representation, but either lack of ability or motivation to carry it through. (Both patients were hospitalized for schizophrenia at the time.)

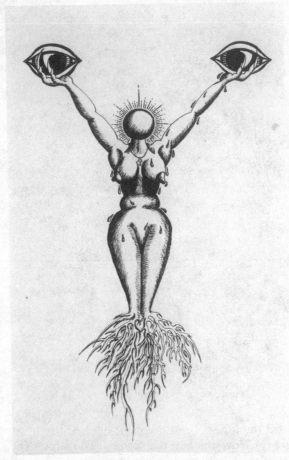

Figure 41. Balance and stability in ink drawing by a schizophrenic young man.

Color

Color can be noted for its amount, variety, intensity, harmony, and so forth. It is often a powerful conveyor of emotion, as in the vivid red paint of Figure 43, the somber gray of Figure 44, or the colorless emptiness of Figure 45. (These patients were all suffering from psychotic depression.)

Line

Most striking in linear quality is the strength or tentativeness of line, its thickness, precision, direction, and amount. Some pictures, such as Fig-

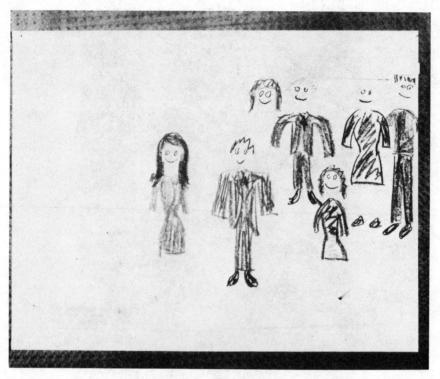

Figure 42. Family portrait.

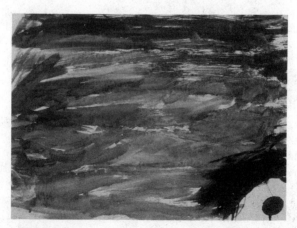

Figure 43. Brilliant red painting by a psychotically depressed young woman.

75

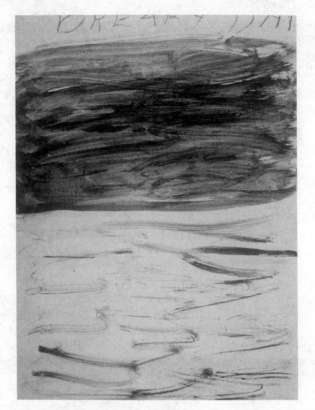

Figure 44. Gray painting by a psychotically depressed young woman.

ure 39, make little use of line. On the other hand, note the difference in linear quality between Figures 35 and 38. The former is spontaneous, the latter planned, controlled, and precise.

Focus or Direction

Does the composition of the picture focus our attention on a particular part that assumes special attention, or is there an all-over pattern? Note the difference between Figure 7 in which the focus is on the central figure who appears to be advancing toward us and Figure 44 where the paper is divided into two portions of light and dark with no central object. On the basis of the pictorial evidence alone we notice a focused image in the former and a more diffuse experience in the latter. In fact, Figure 7

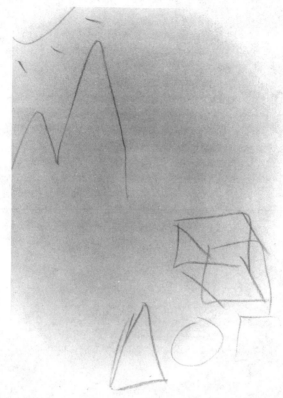

Figure 45. Colorless drawing by a psychotically depressed young man.

represents a "big black man, maybe a killer" following the patient, whereas Figure 44 illustrates another patient's feeling of depression. The former depicts a specific experience, the latter a nonspecific feeling state.

Motion

Stasis versus a feeling of motion sometimes tells us something about a picture's creator. For example, the foliage in Figure 46 appears to hang in space. Nothing is happening in the picture. One might infer that the patient who drew it was rather shut down at the time. Figure 47, on the other hand, is full of action, and we might gather that the patient was quite activated. (Both were hospitalized for psychotic depression.)

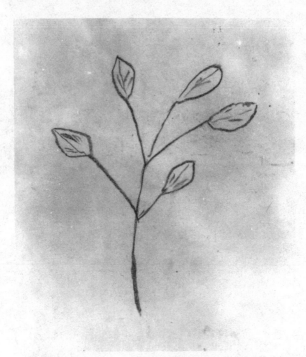

Figure 46. Stasis in a depressed woman's picture.

Detail

Detail, of course, is related to organization and investment of effort. The tight organization and meticulous detailing in Figure 38 indicate a need for control, almost to the point of compulsivity. Figure 37, on the other hand, has so little detail or elaboration that it is evident that the patient was little interested in making the picture, probably due to preoccupation with other things, lack of energy, or lack of motivation.

Texture may provide further elaboration, but it is seldom a prominent consideration in two-dimensional work in art therapy where relatively simple media are used.

Content

The specifics of a picture's content often remain unknown without its creator's explanation. For example, I would not know that Figure 39 represents the patient's hallucination of flashing lights going off in the

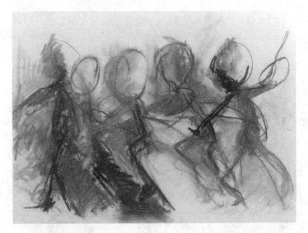

Figure 47. Activity in a depressed woman's picture.

seclusion room if she had not told me so. On the other hand, sometimes content is impactful on the basis of its graphic representation alone. Figure 48 is a bizarre depiction of a person. One can see torment and disturbance in the person portrayed in Figure 49. Figure 50 tells a disturbing story of violence. Observe the sadness expressed in Figure 51. Figure 52 shows incarceration, containment, misery. (All are self-images, the latter

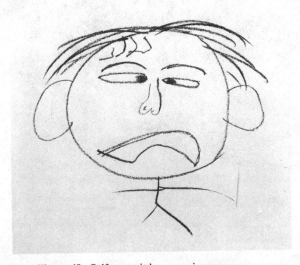

Figure 48. Self-portrait by a manic woman.

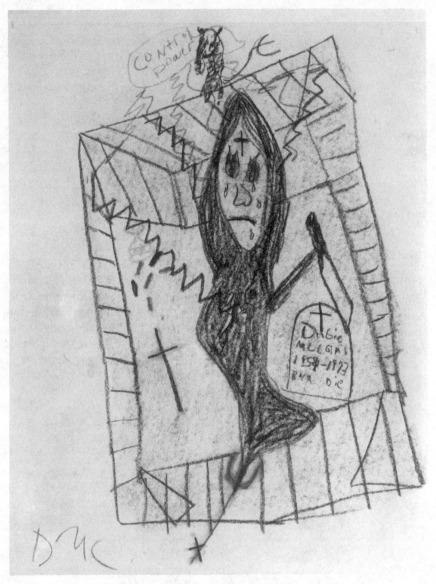

Figure 49. Delusional self-portrait by a schizophrenic young woman.

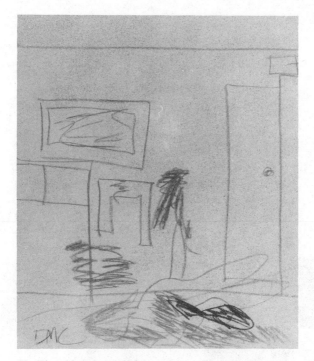

Figure 50. Disturbing story of violence by a schizophrenic young woman.

one by a well-functioning out-patient with an art background, the others by hospitalized psychotics.)

Affect

Sometimes content merges with affect, as in Figure 51. But abstract pictures and nonhuman representations can also express affect. Notice the emptiness of Figure 37, and the whimsey of Figure 34. Lack of affect is also significant, such as in Figure 45 and 38 (which were drawn by the same patient who made Figure 34). Figure 38 appears well-defended, whereas Figure 45 is generally minimal with little investment of feeling or effort.

Investment of Effort

This is a very significant index which art therapists often fail to articulate. When one considers characteristics of art, investment of effort is seldom a

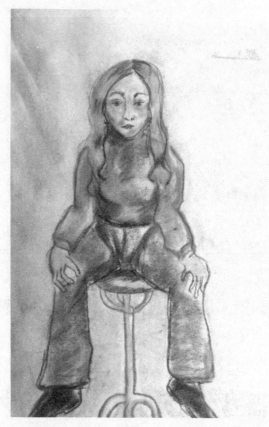

Figure 51. Sadness in a self-portrait by a recovering schizophrenic young woman.

factor because artists are assumed to invest effort in their work. Such is not necessarily the case for art therapy clients for a number of reasons. In the first place, some people are not in art therapy through their own choice and may be resistant to participating (see Chapter 3). Some may be resistant to the whole treatment process. Others may be momentarily resistant due to the pain evoked by the therapy at that time.

In addition to resistance, minimal investment in art-making may result from certain psychiatric and physical conditions. Psychotic confusion or depressive lethargy and apathy are examples of the former. Debilitating physical conditions or physical pain can also hinder effort in art-making. Finally, a relatively common phenomenon in art therapy is the fear of

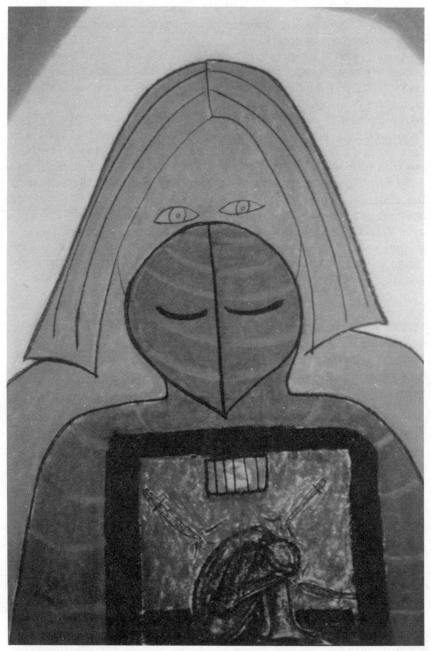

Figure 52. Incarceration in a self-portrait by a well-functioning out-patient.

appearing child-like or a more pervasive feeling of unworthiness leading to awkwardness and discomfort in experimenting with art media for fear of displaying oneself poorly.

As discussed in Chapter 3, part of the effort in art therapy is in helping clients to overcome such inhibitions. Nevertheless, early sessions may be characterized by minimal attempts at art expression as a result of these difficulties and should be recognized as such. The meaningfulness of an art production is clearly determined to a large extent by its creator's investment in it. Figure 37, for example, is easily recognized as a few slap-dash marks on the paper, perhaps to accede to the art therapist's request, but with little of the self put into it. In such cases the art therapist may encourage the patient to understand the feelings present at the time (resistance) or associations to the configuration produced. In other words, the art therapist encourages investing oneself in processing the experience even if investment in actual art-making is minimal. In Figure 41, a contrasting example, it is evident that the patient was invested in communicating a visual message and put time and effort into developing the picture.

SCULPTURAL CHARACTERISTICS

Since the discussions of many of the pictorial characteristics may be applied to comparable sculptural attributes, this section will focus on those characteristics unique to sculpture.

Medium

Most three-dimensional projects involve some sort of building or construction. Although media possibilities are almost limitless, for art therapy purposes, clay is no doubt the most common medium; other frequently used possibilities include wood and plaster.

Clay is a very forgiving medium. It is subject to endless change. Clay's plasticity makes it a particularly apt material for evolving a process and experiencing change. Perhaps more than any other medium, clay invites one to play, to feel, to shape and reshape without necessarily producing a finished object. Its tactile qualities can provoke expression of feeling through pounding, pulling, slapping, breaking, and so forth.

Because of clay's transformative properties, it is often necessary to observe the process of its formation to understand the product. Figure 53

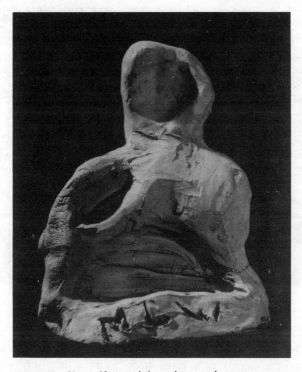

Figure 53. Clay self-portrait by a depressed young woman.

is a self-portrait formed by a depressed young woman who touched on important life experiences in gauging out sections of herself. She was reminded of having exploratory surgery and a kidney removal. Rachel, a middle-aged manic-depressed woman, sculpted two female figures with their arms around each other. She described them as an older woman giving advice to a younger woman. She worked on her figures for several weeks, often positioning me with my arm around her to pose for her sculpture. It was unclear which of us was represented by each figure, as she was a decade older than I, but I was therapist to her. Frequently she gave her figures loving "spankings" with a sculpture tool. Her concentration on this project was remarkable, given her high, often disorganized, manic energy. Clearly, this art product as well as Figure 53 had to be understood as process with observation of the treatment of the clay as an important indicator.

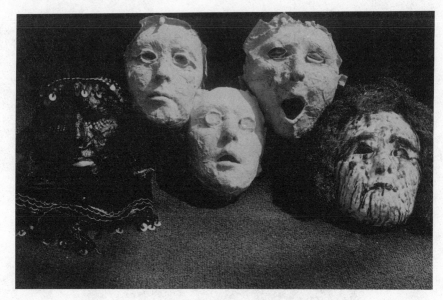

Figure 54. Plaster masks.

Figure 54 is a series of plaster masks, some with shell eyes, made by one person. Plaster may be applied directly to the face or other objects to take their shapes. This series can be recognized as different portraits of the same person, the same face having been used for a mold. One can see the variety in this woman's experience of self. She has taken advantage of the expressive potential of plaster, adding other media such as shells, paint, cloth, wax, and steel wool, to heighten the expressive effects. Would one assume that she is schizophrenic because she views herself so differently from mask to mask? A bizarre self-portrait does not a schizophrenic make. At least I hope that is the case: I made the masks.

Wood, of course, is most often used for construction. Hammering and nailing can offer a release of energy. Woodwork usually requires planning and is often a less personal form of expression than may be possible in clay and plaster.

All these media are used for craft projects as well as art expression. Perhaps the often blurred distinction centers around personal expression. Following another's plan or using a mold created by another is not a personal expression and more readily falls into the category of craft project.

Size

Although size is a significant variable in two-dimensional art, in art therapy it is often influenced by the size of the surface (paper, canvas) available. In three-dimensional projects, on the other hand, size is more likely determined by the creator. A large piece may be impressive, even overwhelming. A small one may be delicate or tentative.

Utility

Some three-dimensional objects are made to serve a purpose, such as a bowl, or a mask that is meant to be worn, or a box. How well it serves its purpose gives information. Clearly the masks in Figure 54 are not meant to be worn (one would be unable to see). They are meant to hang on a wall, and that purpose has been served.

Construction

Gravity exerts an influence in three-dimensional works. For example, a depressed woman tried to mold a clay piece into her daughter ballet dancing. She ended up depicting her seated, with her tutu forming the gravational base. The frail little legs she gave her could not hold her up and they protruded helplessly in front of the figure. In viewing it one could see that a solution was found, but the effect is one of inadequacy. Though this woman was suicidally depressed, she tried to put a pleasant face on all her expressions, both verbally and in her art.

Use of Space: Mass, Negative Space

Figure 53 is a good example of use of negative space. The gauged-out parts give the composition its powerful impact. Treatment of mass can be delicate, heavy, balanced, unbalanced, and so forth. It is a significant expressive component and may tell us something of its author's feeling state.

Soundness of Structure, Permanence

Some pieces are made as sketches or as impermanent experiments. Soundness of structure may tell us of the maker's intentions. In some cases it is evident that a piece is a failed attempt. Children, particularly, may plan projects poorly and become frustrated when materials don't hold together or stand up. Three-dimensional activities are likely to require some technical assistance or instruction from the art therapist.

Texture

Texture is an expressive dimension. Note the gauge marks in Figure 53. One can almost see the artist's hand at work and get some feeling for the tactile nature of the intensity of her experience in the gauging of the clay.

Focus or direction, motion, detail, content, affect, and investment of effort are not discussed further here, as similar considerations apply to these characteristics for two and three-dimensional art works.

COMPARING ART PRODUCTS

The foregoing discussion is applicable to viewing any one piece of art. When there are more than one from a particular individual, it is possible to compare. Changes in style or content can be informative. For example, one piece might be tightly organized and another chaotic. One may be colorful, another devoid of color, to cite extremes. One may depict a desolate landscape, another may show people in close proximity to one another. Change in media can be informative too. A patient may make minimal, empty expressions in whatever medium is used or perhaps a new medium will stimulate a more invested and fuller effort. Wherever possible, therefore, the art therapist can gain a much more complete picture of the patient by viewing as many samples of the patient's art as she can.

Figures 39 and 51 were created by the same young woman (diagnosed acute schizophrenic). Figure 39 was painted in watercolors, and Figure 51 was drawn with pastels. The former is rather formless and flowing, whereas the latter shows well-drawn objects. The patient has utilized each medium effectively to achieve her purposes. In the first she illustrated "lights going off in my head" while confined in the seclusion room. The flow of the paints represents well the indefiniteness of lights, and the colors merge in beautiful blues and golds. In the second picture pastels have been used to draw a self-portrait, expressing the sadness she was feeling. Rather than being limited by an habitual approach, this patient illustrated her flexibility, resourcefulness, and creativity—considerable strengths, to be sure.

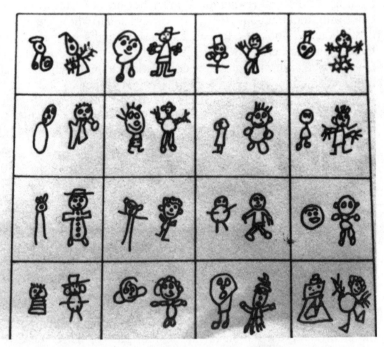

Figure 55. Each block shows two figure drawings by the same child in the course of one week (From Kellogg, R.: *Understanding Children's Art,* by permission of Mayfield Publishing Co., Palo Alto, copyright © 1969, 1970).

One of the best examples I have seen to underscore the importance of looking at a series of art productions is provided by Rhoda Kellogg in *Understanding Children's Art* (1969, 1970). Figure 55, reproduced from her book, shows figure drawings with each block containing two figures made by the same young child in the course of only one week. Such drawings are frequently used to determine a child's mental age. As is apparent from these drawings, the same children tested out at different ages in terms of years within only a few days. It's frightening to realize that consequential decisions, such as institutionalization, are sometimes made on the basis of intelligence tests using a single figure drawing.

Finally, it is important to reiterate that the graphic and sculptural characteristics presented here are the ingredients of the cake. When we take a bite, we don't taste flour, butter, sugar, milk, eggs. Just as the cake is more than the sum of its ingredients, so the art comes from the creative oven as a whole. Art therapists must be receptive to its unique flavor while still understanding that more or less sugar will make a difference.

Let's take a look at a few art expressions and see what we can determine about their creators from the visual expression alone. The pictures I have chosen to discuss are three contrasting examples about which I have little information. All are drawn on 18″ x 24″ paper.

Figure 56 is drawn in black pastel with no color used. Its author has given it a title, otherwise we might not know it is a house. It looks more like a box with little possibility for entrance or egress. It is a stark, minimal drawing, though apparently drawn with some assurance, as the lines are strong and definite, rather than being faint or tentative. The widely-spaced square windows look empty. The object is centered on the paper and is relatively large. The small form at the bottom is probably meant to be a door. This drawing gives the impression of a minimal effort although the drawer probably had sufficient energy to do more (quality of line). The emptiness of the picture as a whole, the empty windows, questionable door, and lack of color all contribute to a lack of affect expressed. One might therefore expect the picture's creator to be rather deadened to feelings or to be holding them back. The minimal effort could be the result of preoccupation, resistance, or depressive lethargy (despite mustering the energy to make definite lines). Most striking, however, is the bizarre representation of the door or lack of it. A house is such a conventional object, stereotypically drawn with a door, a window on either side, a peaked roof, and sometimes a chimney, that this house is

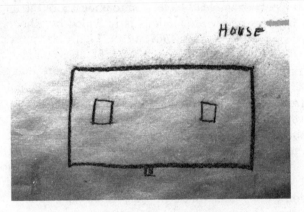

Figure 56. Minimal drawing.

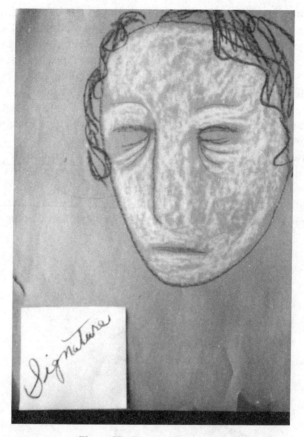

Figure 57. Expressive drawing.

noteworthy in its departure from the norm. Obviously, the depiction here is not a creative attempt at originality. It appears that the drawer attempted a door but could not place it properly and made it very small. We might hypothesize, therefore, that the patient suffered some sort of perceptual distortion. Such could be due either to brain damage or emotional disturbance.

Figure 57 is much more expressive. It is drawn in black pastel on manila paper with the face colored with white and the hair drawn in brown. Like Figure 56, a single object floats in space. The face is not centered but is balanced by the patient's signature. Most noteworthy is the pained expression, the grim mouth, the unseeing eyes. This picture appears to be much more purposeful than Figure 56, with an intention of expressing painful feelings. The patient seems very capable of conveying feelings graphically. Using white pastel and an economy of lines, its creator has produced an original, effective, and expressive communication.

Figure 58 is still another kind of drawing. Unlike the previous two examples, the patient here has used a fuller range of colors. The rose is red with green foliage; the face is drawn in brown with brown hair; the bird is blue; the mountains are drawn in brown with green foreground; the sun is yellow, and there is blue in the sky. This picture is different from the other two also in that numerous objects are depicted rather than having the single focus of the others. None of the three contains a groundline or environment in which the objects reside. All the objects in Figure 58 are well-drawn with sufficient completeness and development to convey an investment of interest and effort by their creator. Compositionally,

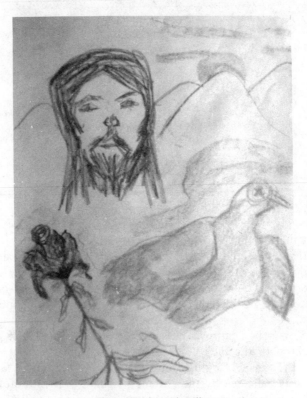

Figure 58. Intentionality.

they fit well on the paper, evidencing planning in use of space. We are left to wonder, however, what the meaningful relationship is among these varied objects. The picture gives the impression that its creator was trying to tell some sort of story. Without an explanation, however, we are left with little understanding of its meaning. Nevertheless, there appears to be intentionality on the part of its creator, as evidenced by the care given the drawing of each object and the well-planned spatial organization.

In viewing all of these art expressions, it is important to keep in mind that they were made in art therapy sessions, usually lasting no more than an hour including discussion time, for the purpose of therapy rather than to produce "art." Therefore, it is necessary to understand them in that context rather than to compare them with work produced in art classes or for the purpose of making "art." Much more effort and planning are likely to go into the latter, rather than the more spontaneous self-expression of an art therapy session. It is with a very different understanding of the context and purpose of art for therapy that we view and comprehend these art expressions compared to the criteria of an art critic appraising art.

DIAGNOSIS

It is evident from the examples presented that although the graphic and sculptural characteristics can provide information about the art therapy client's state, patients of the same diagnosis may exhibit different graphic or sculptural characteristics, as exemplified in the examples in discussions of color, form, focus, motion, and so forth. Nevertheless, the literature is replete with statements such as:

"Schizophrenics make fragmented pictures."
"Depressives make dark pictures."
"Alcoholics frequently draw water."

Although the thrust of this chapter has been the ellucidation of understanding of visual expression, it also makes clear what the limitations are. There is no such thing as a "schizophrenic picture." There are confused looking pictures, fragmented organization, bizarre representations.

Perhaps the point will be made more emphatically if you try your own hand at diagnosis from artwork alone. Take a look at the pictures in Figures 59 and 60. (All the colors are appropriate and probably would not "color" your judgments.) Take a piece of paper and jot down your deter-

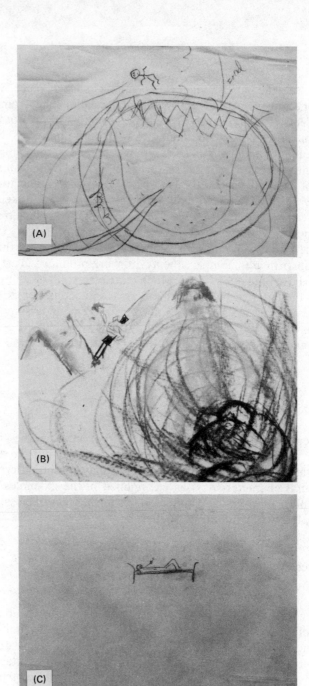

Figure 59. Can you judge psychosis?

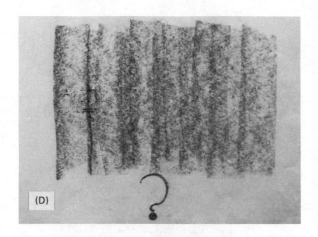

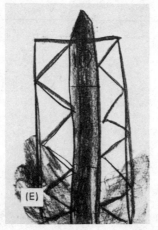

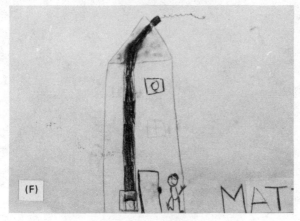

Figure 59. (*Continued*)

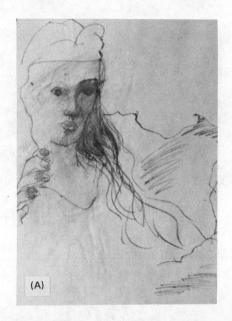

(A)

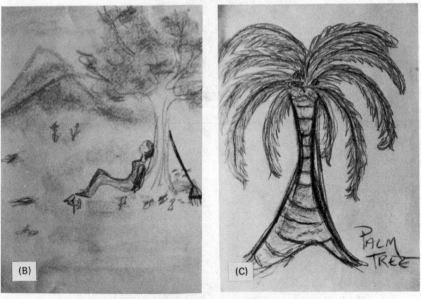

(B)

(C)

PALM TREE

Figure 60. Can you judge psychosis?

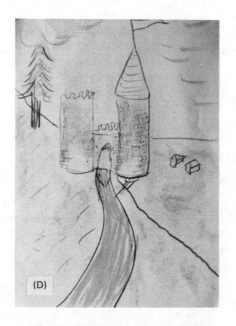

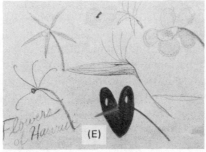

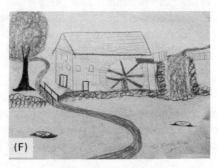

Figure 60. (*Continued*)

minations of which ones were made by psychotic patients. If you can make a more precise diagnosis, add that to your notes. Now I'll give you a bit more information about age and sex to help you out with your evaluation:

Picture 59A: Woman, early 30s
Picture 59B: Woman, mid 40s
Picture 59C: Man, early 30s
Picture 59D: Man, 20s
Picture 59E: Boy, six
Picture 59F: Boy, six
Picture 60A: Woman, early 20s
Picture 60B: Woman, early 20s
Picture 60C: Woman, early 20s
Picture 60D: Man, early 20s
Picture 60E: Man, mid 50s
Picture 60F: Man, mid 40s

Did age and sex help? If so, amend your notations. For answers, see box at the end of this chapter.

Diagnostic labels are consequential not only because they become a permanent part of a patient's record and may influence such treatment decisions as medication, forced hospitalization, and so forth, but they also provide a framework for the therapist's conceptualization about the patient. Therefore, if one assumes that depiction of eyes indicates paranoia and a patient is so labeled on the basis of a drawing, the art therapist may assume that much of the patient's utterances may be paranoid delusions. As a result, if the patient claims that his partner is swindling him, the art therapist may not believe him, even though what he says may be true. A more common occurrence I have witnessed has been staff disbelief of the physical complaints of patients hospitalized for psychotic depression.

It is necessary to be cautious and clear in diagnosis. (Patient assessment is discussed further in Chapter 7 on beginning treatment.) The artwork in conjunction with its meaning to the patient can provide abundant data. The artwork alone, however, usually requires additional information for the unravelling of its meaning.

INFORMATION THAT AIDS UNDERSTANDING
OF ART EXPRESSION

It is important that art therapists and others who attempt to read art expressions know something of an artistic alphabet. Although much can be learned through visual communication, sensitivity to graphic and sculptural characteristics is but a first step in understanding art therapy expressions. To be discussed further are the next steps in enlarging understanding and developing the route toward advancing the therapy.

Many people look on art expressions as windows to the psychic interior. Particularly those who adhere closely to a theoretical and treatment paradigm that emphasizes interpretation may find evidence to support their suppositions. For example, some years ago I volunteered for a demonstration of sand tray work by a prominent Jungian analyst. The event was a meeting of the local Jungian society. After a brief introduction, the analyst instructed another woman and myself to use our sand trays. She built a mountain with a road and put little toy cars on it. Being an art person, I sculpted the sand, mixing it with water and adding shells and stones to make a rather bizarre-looking face with strange eyes. The Jungian audience gasped, "She's made Cassandra." Cassandra was blind but had psychic vision. My sand face was very moving to me, having a particular connection to a painful circumstance in my life. The eyes as well as other aspects of the face were especially expressive of my situation. The Cassandra myth was not particularly relevant to my personal connection with this spontaneous and unplanned representation. The point I am making here is that interpretation that is not centered in the art-maker's experience may actually interfere with one's more accurate understanding of the art. It may also inhibit the therapeutic process in dividing therapist from client.

Just as the art may speak to the observer without resort to speculative leaps, so it is possible to utilize other information to enhance understanding. The first source is an obvious one. If the art therapist has been working with the client for a period of time, she may already be familiar with the client's visual language. Many people use repeated symbols or colors to represent particular experiences or feelings. One patient with whom I worked, for example, associated purple with her mother. Another repeatedly represented her husband with the Star of David. His name was David and they both were Jewish. Clients have often told me of their association of colors to particular feelings. As is obvious, these symbols and associations are idiosyncratic and not necessarily universal. Therefore, it is important to know what the meaning holds for the client rather than to assume particular meanings. One patient, for example, used blue to represent death, another intellect, another spirit, and still another cold.

A frequent source of information is a patient's records. Some art therapists, however, prefer to see a patient initially free of influence from colleagues' assessments. I prefer to work this way in order to respond to the client without bias. All too frequently, we find what we are expecting to see. For example, if the chart tells us that the patient has been alcoholic for many years, we may find indices of organicity in the drawings that we would not have noticed otherwise. I prefer the opposite route, one in which the art informs me of the problem rather than my finding a questionable confirmation in the art.

Figure 61 is such an example. It was drawn by an intelligent middle-aged woman. She was hospitalized for depression. In the art therapy session, she became frustrated with her drawing because she could not "make the lake lie down." She was very much aware that her picture was not "right," and I was surprised that, try as she would, her lake would not "lie down" for her. I suspected brain damage. Later it was discovered that she had been a secret alcoholic for years. This example illustrates that had the patient been given technical assistance by an art therapist in this instance, valuable diagnostic information might have been lost.

Years ago when art therapy was much less sophisticated than it is today, I read an account that so startled me I remember it now, 20 years

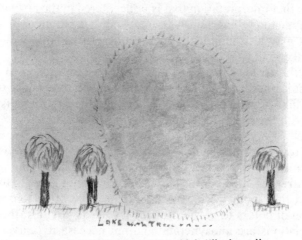

Figure 61. The lake that wouldn't "lie down."

later. The report was about a confused foreign-born patient who co_
speak English. No one in the hospital spoke his language so there was
very little information in his record. The one item known about his background was that his family of origin was composed of five people. In art
therapy he drew a picture with four trees. The art therapist assumed that
they represented his other family members.

This is an extreme example of undue influence from a record. Sometimes information gained in art therapy disputes a patient's record. For
example, the chart of a recently hospitalized young man diagnosed schizophrenic indicated that he was no longer delusional. Yet when I saw him
in art therapy his pictures indicated the possibility of remaining delusions,
and his responses to some exploratory questions confirmed it. There are
many instances, of course, where information from the patient's records
provides valuable clarification, such as a recent suicide attempt or a significant loss. Staff conferences and communications from other staff
members furnish similar background data.

CHILD SEXUAL ABUSE

An area in which determinations from drawings are particularly prominent is sexual abuse of children. Child sexual abuse is a problem that has
received considerable professional attention as well as media focus in
recent years. Art therapists are especially interested in this area because
many professionals believe that evidence of this trauma, that is apparently more prevalent than was recognized until recently, may be found in
the drawings of young children. These victims are often unable to produce
reliable evidence verbally for both developmental and emotional reasons,
and extended questioning is often added stress to what is already a harm-
ful situation for the child.

If art expression were able to provide the needed information for assessment, prevention, treatment, and legal purposes, many difficulties
inherent in this situation could be handled more readily. Unfortunately, as
is found in other areas utilizing art for assessment, the solutions are not so
simple. Art therapists engaged in systematic study of pictorial symbols
hypothesized to be associated with sexual abuse have not discovered
conclusive relationships (Cohen, 1985; Siden, 1985). On the other hand,
art therapists are seeking to capitalize on the interest in this subject (Wohl
& Kaufman, 1985).

The following are examples that illustrate a variety of communications

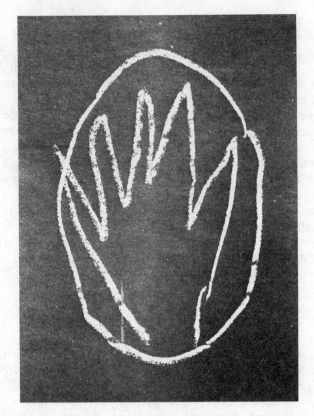

Figure 62. "Daddy's hand on my vagina."

related to possible sexual abuse and the ways in which the art therapist may understand them.*

Figure 62 was drawn by a six-year-old girl. When brought to a staff meeting, the picture was identified by one staff member as "A tulip in an egg." The child described the picture as "Daddy's hand on my vagina." In this instance, although the picture is not specific, the child's comments are, and no speculation is necessary. The picture prompted the child to discuss her experience of sexual abuse.

Figure 63 is pictorially more explicit. Children in a kindergarten class were given a cut-out house and asked to draw their families. Johnny drew

---

* These clients were treated at C.A.U.S.E.S., the child abuse unit of Illinois Masonic Hospital, by Jean Vanderlinde.

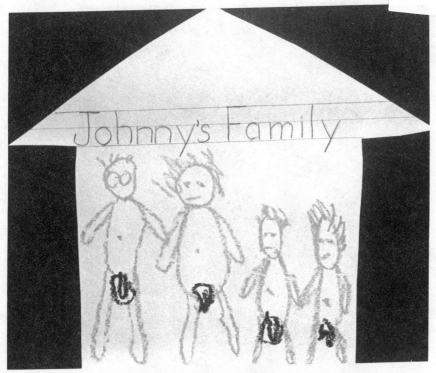

Figure 63. Picture from kindergarten.

his family in green with pronounced red genitals. The teacher displayed the children's pictures at a PTA meeting, and Johnny's parents became alarmed and sought consultation. Does the picture's focus on large red genitals indicate sexual abuse? We do not know from pictorial evidence alone. The most we can say is that there is a preoccupation with the genital area. Further information is required to determine what this means to the child.

Figure 64 is the Easter Bunny drawn by a six-year-old girl. Unlike Figure 63 or even Figure 62, once we know its meaning, there is no explicit depiction of genitalia. In this case, it was the process of the drawing that was informative. When the child came to the lower torso, she asked the therapist to color it. The therapist said, "That's a special area, isn't it?" The child agreed and then as the therapist colored the genital area, the child described what happened to her "down there," fondling by her father.

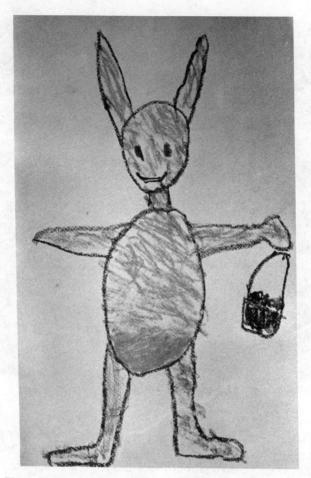

Figure 64. Easter Bunny: Therapist was asked to color lower torso.

Finally, Figure 65 was drawn by an almost mute eight-year-old girl. She was known to have been raped by her step-father. She said nothing about her picture and we can only speculate that the object represents genitalia. The upside-down look of the object may be due to the child's lack of familiarity with male sexual organs or may be congruous with her experience of the rape. Lowenfeld and Brittain (1970) write that children draw what they experience rather than what they see.

As these examples illustrate, sexually related imagery by young children does not necessarily indicate sexual abuse. During early childhood

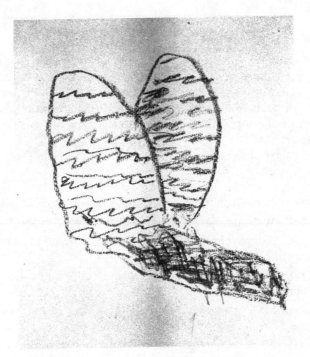

Figure 65. Picture by raped eight-year-old girl.

there can be an expectable and healthy interest in sexual differences. Concerns about sex expressed in images can be very useful for the explorations of these issues, whether they involve ordinary interest, problematic preoccupation, or experience of sexual abuse.

CONCLUSION

The most complete and reliable source of information about the art comes from the client or patient. As stated previously, two of the most important aspects of the art therapists' interactions with her clients are the encouragement of art expression and its creative exploration. It is through the latter that clients and art therapist discover together the import of the art for the client. Because this is such an important function in the art therapist's advancement of the therapeutic process, it is discussed in a separate chapter to follow.

Answers to Diagnostic Quiz

Do all the pictures in Figure 59 look as though they were made by psychotics, and all those in Figure 60 by nonpsychotics? If that was your judgment, you were 100 percent—wrong! But don't feel too badly; I selected the pictures to throw you off in order to emphasize the point that it is difficult, if not impossible, to make diagnostic determinations on the basis of the art alone.

The particulars of the people who made the pictures in Figures 59 and 60 are as follows:

Picture 59A: Nonpsychotic obese woman in out-patient treatment

Picture 59B: Well-functioning art therapist (nonpatient)

Picture 59C: Nonpsychotic alcoholic man in out-patient alcohol treatment program

Picture 59D: Nonpsychotic alcoholic man in out-patient alcohol treatment program

Picture 59E: Six-year-old nonpsychotic MBD boy in out-patient treatment

Picture 59F: Six-year-old well functioning boy (nonpatient)

Picture 60A: Hospitalized schizophrenic young woman, acute phase, nonmedicated

Picture 60B: Hospitalized schizophrenic young woman, acute phase, nonmedicated

Picture 60C: Suicidal young woman hospitalized for psychotic depression; suicided a month after making picture

Picture 60D: Hospitalized schizophrenic young man, acute phase, nonmedicated

Picture 60E: Suicidal middle-aged man hospitalized for bipolar affective psychosis, manic phase; eventually suicided

Picture 60F: Hospitalized manic-depressed man, manic phase

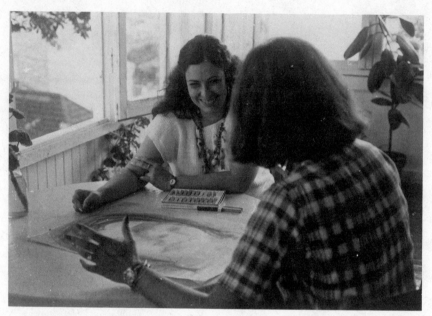

Figure 66. Art therapist Barbara Fish with a client in an individual art therapy session.

CHAPTER 5

Relating to Clients Around Art Expression

As stated previously, the art therapist's effort is a two-stage process: the encouragement of art expression and the exploration of the art expression. Chapter 3 focuses on the former. This chapter discusses how the art therapist relates to the art and to the client in relation to the art. The chapter begins with the nuts and bolts operations around relating to the art, continues with goals and methods of creating a therapeutic alliance and understanding transference phenomena in art therapy, proceeds to a discussion of the art therapeutic relationship within noninsight oriented populations, and concludes with a look at making art with clients.

The art is an expression of the client, so it is treated as such. It is taken seriously and respected. The art therapist does not invade it, either physically by working on it* or verbally with unfounded interpretation. If it is necessary for her to handle it, she does so with care. Because the art's value is in its representative quality of the client, the art therapist does not try to influence its direction. In order that it be truly the client's, she does not interfere in its development. Her position in relation to the art is one of acceptance and interest, not judgment. Nor does she make *a priori* assumptions about it (Chapter 4). Rather, she is open and attentive.

OBSERVING THE ART-MAKING

Processing the art with the client proceeds as follows: Having encouraged the client to engage in artwork (Chapter 3), the art therapist has now moved to the next step. She observes the client working because the way the art develops is often very telling. A client may change the object considerably. For example, Figure 67, made by a six-year-old boy, underwent a number of transformations before it was smeared over in disgust.

---

* Exceptions are discussed at the end of the chapter.

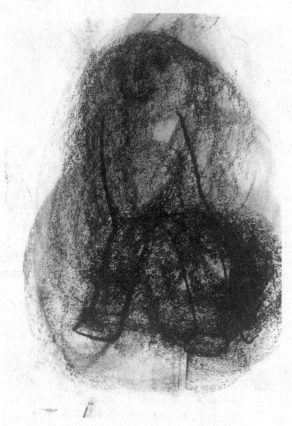

Figure 67. Drawing by a six-year-old boy that changed many times before being smeared over.

In addition to changes, there are other important actions to observe as well. In Figure 68, drawn by a middle-aged man hospitalized for psychotic depression, the trees in the lower part of the picture were drawn from left to right with soft pencil. As he progressed, his pencil strokes became more and more forceful. In response to my comment that a picture is a safe place to ventilate any anger he might be feeling, he bore down heavily on the pencil blackening the semi-circular road by going over it again and again. This patient communicated very little verbally, nor does the subject matter of the picture, a view from my office window, offer much. After drawing the road, he seemed exhausted, crumpled into a chair, and withdrew into himself, saying nothing more. Three days later, he killed

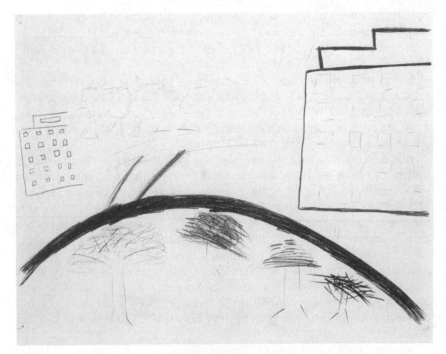

Figure 68. Progressive forcefulness in pencil strokes by a suicidal man.

himself. No one on the staff had suspected he was suicidal. His most revealing communication was the manner in which he drew this picture and reacted to it. (This patient was one of my first [over two decades ago]. Had this session occurred today, I would have pursued the problem with the patient and the staff more thoroughly.)

In most instances I would not interrupt the client's concentration in the art-making process. If he wishes to talk, I listen and respond, but do not try to extend conversation. If the session is almost over and the client is still working, I might suggest stopping so that we may have time to reflect together on the work. I tell the client that the art can be finished next session or I provide materials for work between sessions.

DISCUSSING THE ART

Once the artwork is obviously completed, I wait expectantly for the client to tell me about it. In early sessions I ask the client to discuss the work, but after a while he knows what to expect and it is not necessary for me to invite discussion. By waiting, I try to convey the idea that the art therapy is the client's, just as the artwork is, and I want him to take responsibility for its direction.

Under most circumstances the client says something about the art. The art therapist may ask a few questions that don't lead to anything special, and may feel baffled about where to go from there. Although it takes experience to become adept at helping clients to explore their art, there are some approaches that may be helpful.

It is important to wait to hear what the client will say. It is also important not to rush the client or convey the notion that one must come up with a meaning. By allowing the client to explore at will, the direction and areas of interest will be the client's rather than the therapist's. Only after the client has completed this tack should the art therapist enter in. She may ask some questions for her own clarification, either about the art or what the client has said. For example, if there is an unexplained object in a picture, or if the client has referred to a color and she is not sure which one, or a person or event that she cannot identify, then she would request clarification. Also, she would want to know the client's intention if he had one (e.g., that he was trying to portray his childhood home, not just any house).

Where she goes from there is perhaps the point requiring the most skill, sensitivity, and insight in art therapy. The options are innumerable. Often the choice is one of responding to what has been presented or to encourage the client to explore further, although her response may have the effect of doing both at once. She might react to the feeling level of the communication, such as "That must have been a very painful experience." Sometimes people use the art as a springboard to discussion and move far from the original image. I usually bring them back to the art expression eventually because I believe there are relationships between the image and where it leads even when the latter seems far-a-field. I might ask about something the client is saying, such as "Is that feeling expressed in your picture?"

In moving a client to explore further, there are many possibilities. The feeling dimension of the expression is usually significant. I might ask about the mood of the representation, or how the client felt while creating it, or the feelings now in looking at it. Less often I would comment on the feelings expressed by saying something like "That face certainly looks angry." I would more likely ask the client what sort of expression the face has. The reason is the same as mentioned previously, not to impose an assumption or interpretation, but to encourage the client to explore and interpret.

Some of the other possibilities include encouragement toward free association, comparison with other art the client has made, telling a story about the artwork, imagining what it would be like to be a person or object represented, dramatizing elements in the art, and so forth. It is difficult to innumerate all the possibilities because they are the art therapist's responses to what is presented rather than routines that are planned in advance. This is yet another area where the art therapist's creativity comes into play.

How does the art therapist decide what are the important directions to take, when to question or suggest, and when to be silent and wait for the client to take the initiative? The answer, of course, is the stuff of which clinical judgment is made. But in general, the art therapist can be guided by several principles. Her intent is two-fold: to encourage the client's self-processing and to convey that she is interested and supportive. Indications of interest and support are likely to come naturally in an established therapeutic relationship. Early in therapy, however, the client may have doubts and need reassurance. Obviously the art therapist is always genuine in anything she says and does not give false support or reassurance. Early on I make a point of congratulating clients on their good therapeutic work.

In determining what is likely to encourage self-processing, the art therapist must make assessments of such client needs as getting in touch with feelings, examining defenses, exploring fantasy, and so forth. Timing makes a difference. A client is often ready to probe more deeply once trust has been built. The art therapist encourages continuity, relating one element or expression to another, and helping the client to see patterns in his life.

The art therapist is often confronted with a myriad of material: elements in the art expression, how the client has related to them, further associations, feelings expressed and perhaps some suspected but not expressed, the client's behavior, where all this material appears to fit in the ongoing work, and so forth. How, then, does the art therapist decide what to pursue with the client? She looks for therapeutic "pay dirt." That is the material that elicits strong feeling, that gives evidence of demonstrating a pattern, that bears an important relationship to other material that has come up, that may be productive of insight, that is unexpected and therefore may show a new side of things, a change in artistic style that may indicate a change in psychic state, and most importantly, that which intrigues or interests the client.

Naturally, the art therapist cannot always be on target in the direction she pursues. She may have a hunch, question the client about it, and get nowhere. Sometimes her hunch is a good one but the client is not yet ready to deal with the material she is pointing out. It is not a gross error to get no place. If she is sensitive to her client, this won't happen constantly; otherwise the client might be left feeling that the art therapist is completely out of touch.

RESISTANCE

But what does the art therapist do when she is convinced she is on target and the client won't take the path she is pointing out; or worse, when a patient denies any meaning at all to the art; or worse still, does such minimal art that there is hardly anything with which to work? In other words, how does the art therapist handle resistance? She has three choices: she can just let it go and move on to other things, either further discussion, more art-making, or just sitting in silence; she can push the client to follow her original suggestion; or, she can deal with the resistance. I usually find the third option the most productive. So I might say, "This appears to be a difficult area for you to get into. What seems to be getting in the way?" Or if the client has said, "I don't want to talk about that," I might ask, "What do you think would happen if you did?" These questions enable the client to examine fears around self-examination and revelation.

Finally, it is important to realize that as abundant as art expression is in furnishing therapeutic material, no one piece need be plumbed to its ultimate depths. If the client seems to be able to go no further with a particular art expression, it doesn't mean that valuable material will be lost. Whatever is there will surface again and again in future artwork.

THERAPEUTIC ALLIANCE

Throughout the processing of the art expressions the art therapist gives the meta-message that art therapy is a shared journey in which the art therapist accompanies the client on inward and outward paths. Most often the client does the leading, indicating the territories to be explored. Sometimes the art therapist offers guidance or makes observations. The "we're in this together" feeling the art therapist tries to promote is enormously supportive to the client. With a trusted companion one may be willing to venture into dark and shadowy places bringing light to what previously had been too frightening to explore.

Figure 69 is an example of that most interesting time when a psychotic

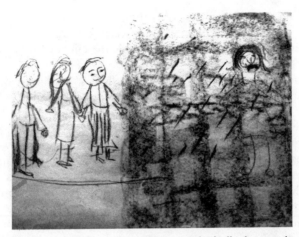

Figure 69. Questioning her delusions by a psychotically depressed woman.

patient is beginning to question delusions. An elderly woman hospitalized for psychotic depression drew that moment when she was unsure what was real and what wasn't. Putting these images on paper, "out there," and sharing them with me took a lot of the terror and confusion out of the chaos this patient was experiencing. The therapeutic alliance that had already been established helped her to sort out her perceptions. Another similarly diagnosed hospitalized woman drew a grid-like structure that had appeared in her soup and frightened her. I suggested that we go to the dining room and investigate. I noticed that the overhead florescent light was covered by such a structure so I put a bowl of water on the table to see if it would catch the reflection. Sure enough, it did. The patient was greatly relieved to discover that the strange look of her soup was reality-based and not a hallucination. Our therapeutic alliance enabled us to become coinvestigators in ferreting out the immediate source of her distress. In a sense, she was able to borrow my reality to make sense of her own perceptions.

Although, in general, the art therapist follows the client's lead and encourages the client to take leadership, there are times when the art therapist provides direction, may interpret, or confront. Decisions about these interventions are governed by the state of the therapeutic alliance and transference ramifications. If the client is strong enough to resist an interpretation that does not fit and to accept one that does, interpretation can be helpful. If in doubt, however, don't. Insight is almost always more powerful when it is reached by the client rather than suggested by the therapist. Too often therapists enjoy their own brilliant insights too much to refrain from leaping to them aloud instead of suggesting a direction to take or an area to explore that would enable the client to come to the same insight himself.

Sometimes I offer an observation to a client by explicitly describing it as my own reaction rather than fact. For example, I might say, "Although this doesn't exactly fit with your description of the picture, to me the face looks angry. Does it look that way to you?" Or, "This may just be my idiosyncratic reaction, but I see a face in that form at the lower left."

There may be times when confrontation is useful. An example is, "I think you're fooling yourself when you portray yourself as a helpless victim." The purpose for doing this is to cause the client to reflect. An argument over who is right is hardly productive. Sometimes the same purpose can be achieved by taking the opposite tack. By emphasizing how victimized the client is, the therapist may help him to see that maybe the situation really isn't as extreme as all that. It is important in this sort of unraveling to encourage the fullest exploration possible. So if the client feels like a victim, the art therapist would promote the expression of those feelings and a reflection on them from many vantage points including past experiences before confronting such a stance.

When the therapeutic alliance is sufficiently strong, humor may have its place as well. If therapist and client can join in amusement at the absurdity of the client's perspectives or behavior, such sharing of feeling is usually experienced by the client as a loving acceptance of his problems. The humor should never be of a mocking nature. If the client mocks himself, the therapist should not join in, but rather point out what he's doing and suggest he take a look at his contemptuous attitude toward himself. In a strong therapeutic alliance there is room for sharing other feelings as well, such as sadness and joy.

The art therapist may remind the client of important directions to take based on her understanding of his problems and treatment goals. For example, if he has trouble recognizing and expressing anger, she may indicate times when he appears to be avoiding dealing with such feelings. I sometimes try to make such difficulties a little easier for clients by saying such things as, "If I had been treated that way, I would be absolutely furious." In this way I try to convey that anger would be a normal and appropriate reaction under the circumstances.

Feelings of anger and disappointment are often very problematic. Clients certainly have difficulty in dealing with anger toward their therapist and with disappointment in her. Therapists frequently have difficulty with these feelings toward clients too. When the therapist suspects such feelings on the part of the client, she should encourage their expression and join the client in supporting the feelings and trying to understand them. The natural reaction to being attacked (as the therapist may be in the client's anger or feel in the client's disappointment) is to become defensive. If she has confidence in her work, she is less likely to erect her defenses. Clients' anger toward the therapist usually results from their feelings of having been let down by her, not cared about, or mistreated in some way. There are usually transference shadows coloring the experience. Nevertheless, it is necessary for the therapist to relate to the feelings in the light of justified grievances first. The client needs to be heard out and responded to at this level before he may be open to looking at his predisposing attitudes. Figure 70 shows a client's anger as a red barrier between the larger bird (me) and the smaller bird (herself), which prevents the smaller bird from being fed properly.

In expressing the negative feelings, the client's meta-message to the therapist is that she is not doing a very good job. The therapist's temptation to justify herself may be strong. If she can resist it and be accepting of the client's feelings, she is more likely to encourage a full expression of feeling for the future rather than to lead the client to believe either that she is too fragile to hear his criticisms of her or that she will retaliate with a withdrawal of her caring, both often expected outcomes on the part of the client. If I feel I have let the client down, I generally offer my appreciation to him for sharing those difficult feelings with me and my apologies or regrets for not having served him better. This sort of sharing usually strengthens our therapeutic relationship.

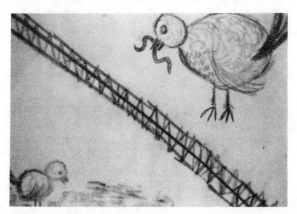

Figure 70. An angry red barrier between client and art therapist by a well functioning outpatient.

I often prepare clients in advance. I tell them I will make them a promise. This usually gets their attention since it's so unusual for anyone to promise results in any kind of treatment. Of course, I don't promise a result. I promise the client that I will disappoint him. I tell him that I will not do so deliberately, but since I am only human there may be moments when I am not sufficiently sensitive to him or when I might be preoccupied with my own concerns. In this way I let him know that I expect perfection neither from myself nor him and that I will be accepting of my own flaws and not unduly upset if he points them out to me. It is often helpful to model self-acceptance in this way.

What about the therapist's anger and disappointment in the client? Regarding the latter, she may be sad if a client who was progressing well backslides, but if she truly believes the therapy belongs to the client, as does his life, she will allow him to lead it has he chooses. Her disappointment is more likely in herself for not doing as good a job as she would wish. In this case, she may need supervision or some personal work on her own self-acceptance or perhaps on her grandiose notions that she can "fix" anyone. Experienced therapists recognize that even with the best of work there are some people who will remain despairing or unable to live in harmony with others.

Anger is another matter. As always, awareness is essential. If a client has been abusive to her, the therapist must let him know firmly what her limits are. She may need to delineate alternatives. But she must be sure her own angry feelings are not the result of countertransference issues. The therapeutic alliance is a training ground for human interaction and as such offers productive experience in the difficult task of handling anger. The therapist models that anger need not be destructive but can be channeled into useful energy for redefining a relationship.

TRANSFERENCE

It is necessary to bear in mind that the therapeutic alliance transpires within the context of the transference relationship and is significantly shaped by it. To loose sight of this phenomenon is to miss most of what is happening in art therapy. The art therapist's interest is usually felt as caring, but it may also be experienced as intrusive. The client's cooperation may be self-exploration or merely an effort to please, based on a lifelong pattern of relationship to authority. Resistance may be fear, shame, anger at the therapist or the institution, once again derived from childhood expectations.

It is helpful to remember that art-making is not a customary activity for most people. Especially initially they are likely to feel awkward. Many are reminded of their elementary school days and feel comparably child-like in relation to an authoritative teacher who must be pleased and obeyed. Although it is important for the art therapist to convey that art therapy is a place for the client to express whatever he wishes, as opposed to school, it is also important to foster an examination of those childlike feelings that are aroused by the art therapy situation.

Beyond these more or less apparent considerations, it is useful to step back and take a broader look at the influence of art-making in therapy and for therapy on the traditional transference relationship. It is also important to recognize that art produced in art therapy is influenced by that particular context of a transference relationship as opposed to art produced elsewhere. In art therapy, both client and art therapist are aware that the art will be used to further the therapeutic process, that its purpose is therapy. To a large extent, the art becomes the meeting place of client and art therapist. These conditions exert a powerful influence on the nature of the art product's development. I'm not suggesting that clients and patients set about to make art that is therapeutic (whatever they may believe that to be), but rather that their expectations around the sort of processing to which it will be subjected and their expectations of the way it will be received by the art therapist are significant determiners of the nature of the art expression.

Against this background are further considerations of how art-making may influence transference phenomena. These include both the person of the art therapist and the process of making art in art therapy. It is also important to consider art therapy's important potential to hold a mirror up to the transference relationship in the form of transference portraits. These portraits may picture transference to the treatment facility and to other staff members, as well as to the art therapist. Art making may also induce some unique countertransference phenomena as well.

The Art Therapist

In considering the person of the art therapist, it is important to recognize that transference is not a random occurrence. Although transference is an unconscious process that may be a part of any human relationship (Moore and Fine, 1968), there are some situations that encourage its development more than others. Those involving authority figures evoking a child to parent sort of transference are the most obvious. In fact, the major thrust of a psychoanalysis is the facilitation and resolution of the "transference neurosis" (Moore & Fine, 1968, p. 92).

When I think of the selectivity involved in transference reactions, the image of a coat hook comes to mind. Certain personal characteristics in particular situations provide convenient hooks on which to hang a transference. The art therapist, by the very nature of her work, furnishes some very accommodating hooks for some heavy transference garments.

An art therapist is a provider. Other therapists certainly provide as well, but in addition to all the intangibles a therapist may give (such as interest, care, attention, insight), art therapists also provide tangible supplies. As mentioned in Chapter 2, the exclamation of an adolescent upon seeing the art materials on her initial visit to my office at the NIH was, "All this for free?" She had been making art for a long time, and to her my office looked life heaven. She hadn't even interacted with me yet, and already I was perceived as the all-giving mother. (Naturally, meager supplies could evoke feelings toward a withholding parent.)

Because the patient or client is called upon to make a product in art therapy and because art-making is not an activity in which most people feel very skilled, the art therapist may readily be experienced as a critical parent, a harsh judge whose approval, the patient believes, will not be forthcoming.

Another parental hook is one-who-knows-the-meaning-of-things. Young children turn to their parents (especially their mothers) to explain things and to make the world comprehensible to them. Art expression often has about it an element of mystery. Patients may suspect that their art has hidden meaning that the art therapist can read to which they themselves are blind. Many clients have requested me to tell them what their pictures mean. This dependency on an all-knowing mother at times even conveys the perception of a sorcerer or god-like being. Expectedly, the power given the art therapist as one who is nurturing and all-knowing evokes negative feelings as unrealistic dependency needs are inevitably frustrated.

Occasionally, a patient treated by a variety of staff in a treatment facility may find in the art therapist a messenger-type transference hook. This might be particularly likely for people who have communicated through one parent to another. The art therapist readily becomes a "messenger" because the art product is such a tangible message.

Figure 71 is an example of such a transference relation to her psychiatrist by a hospitalized manic-depressive woman who was very angry at him because she felt he underestimated her abilities. Underneath the anger were painful feelings associated with his confirmation of her own

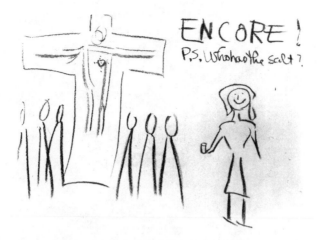

Figure 71. Anger at her psychiatrist who is here crucified, drawn by a manic woman.

self doubts. She had been militantly religious, but at this time felt extremely disappointed about not being "saved." She drew Jesus crucified with bullet-holes in the shape of a cross shot in his heart. Beside him is herself, smiling and holding a salt shaker. She said she would like to crucify Jesus again, shoot bullets through his heart and pour salt in the wounds. She joked about "twisting off Jesus' penis." Then, amidst sobs, angry outbursts, and sarcastic glee, she said her revenge on her psychiatrist would be "to twist off his peter, but I really don't think he has one." There is a clear connection in her rage at her doctor, Jesus, the neglectful husband she divorced, and her alcoholic father—all men whom she felt cared for her inadequately.

In this example the art therapist (myself) was probably used as a messenger to convey the patient's anger to her psychiatrist. But to consider this picture as serving only that purpose is to miss its obvious facilitation of ventilation of feeling with the concommitant opportunity for exploring those feelings through imagistic metaphor and sharing them with another (the art therapist). In this case, such communication was probably easier than dealing directly with the psychiatrist.

The Art-Making Process

As noted earlier, the person of the art therapist, by the nature of her work, may readily evoke certain transference projections. But beyond that, the

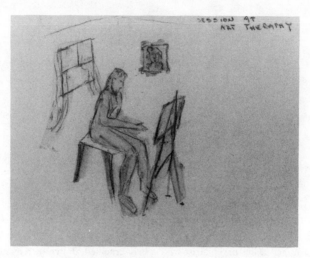

Figure 72. Vulnerability in art therapy.

process of art-making in art therapy sessions may also stir up old familiar feelings or patterns of behavior in the way a client relates to the art therapist.

Although people undergoing any sort of psychotherapy often feel exposed, they may feel particularly vulnerable around the unexpected aspects of themselves that are sometimes revealed in their art. Figure 72 is an especially clear representation of these feelings accompanied by sexual overtones. A middle-aged man hospitalized for anxiety and depression had intended to depict Rodin's "The Thinker" but instead produced a picture of himself nude, working at an easel with my head gazing at him from a framed picture on the wall. He titled the painting "Session at Art Therapy." In the picture, he is revealed naked to me, while I am "safely ensconced in a frame" and have no body. He explained that this way I could not be "active." The lack of mutuality in this situation is one in which the patient may feel exposed, evaluated, and judged in producing a product which may be self-revealing in ways the patient feels unable to control.

Many of those who come to art therapy have not participated in art activities since childhood. As mentioned previously, often they feel thrown back to school days. Some enjoy the regressive feelings stimulated by the art materials, but many are embarrassed by what they consider the child-like appearance of their work. The regressive nature of artwork for those unaccustomed to it sometimes leaves art therapy clients feeling deskilled and ineffectual. This aspect of transference to the process is usually readily overcome with the help of a sensitive art therapist.

In group therapy there is an expectable sibling-like rivalry for the attention of the therapist, but in group art therapy it may take on the added dimension of encouraging art that will interest the therapist and help to establish a position among peers.

When I have encouraged patients to try out the art materials, they have sometimes responded initially by indicating that they were making a picture "for" me. They have viewed the art as an activity and product I wanted rather than as something they were doing for themselves. They behaved like cooperative, obedient children trying to please mommie or teacher.

Transference to the Institution

Since the art products provide an especially clear, dramatic, and revealing reflection of transference phenomena, they may refract various facets of the transference. Figure 73, a depiction of life on the ward drawn by a schizophrenic patient, illustrates aspects of transference to the institution in the eye looking through the seclusion room window, the barred window of the seclusion room, the rushing doctor, pharmocological mood determinants, as well as the anger and sadness she was feeling. Although feelings of being abused or neglected in this sort of milieu may be reality-based, they may also be rooted in early family experience in which the patient felt helpless and of little importance.

Countertransference

It is easier for therapists to discuss and illustrate transference than it is to look at countertransference. Nevertheless, the art therapy may evoke some unique countertransference phenomena as well. We may enter the mode of art teacher or achievement-oriented parent and encourage clients and patients to produce "good art," sometimes at the expense of a larger acceptance of whatever they do or their own self-determination. In this way, our needs for perfection or to control may collude with the helpless quality of a patient's transference. Seldom do we do this overtly. It is much more likely to be a subtle influence through which the patient comes to see where our interests lie.

When I first entered the field I read a very interesting book on working with groups of retarded individuals through art. If I had not looked at the book's pictures I would have been enthralled with the work. The draw-

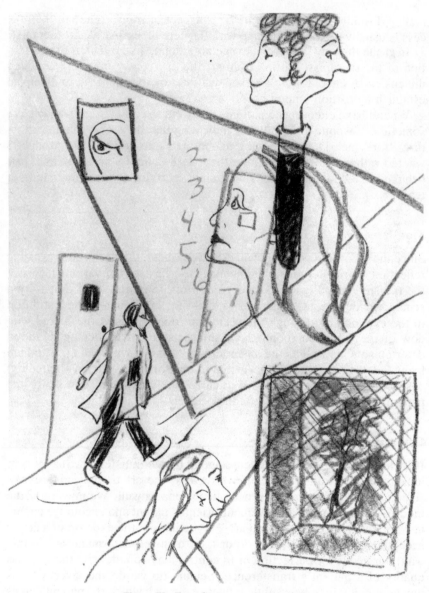

Figure 73. Transference to the hospital.

ings told a story quite different from the impressive words. The pictures were charming, to be sure, with a unique distinctive style. But they all looked almost exactly alike! Somehow, the clients were not being encouraged toward self-expression, but rather toward copying a particular model. Just as the art therapist should encourage self-direction in life choices, rather than using therapy as an instrument to ensure social conformity, so should she encourage self-determination and expression in the art. Some who have a strong commitment to aesthetics may do otherwise and impose their artistic values on their clients. Just as therapists who have convictions as to how the clients should behave may give the message that they are not alright as they are, so the art therapist may convey that a client's visual self-expression is not acceptable without "corrections." When this sort of nonacceptance occurs, the art therapist should suspect countertransference problems.

Because we treasure the art-making process and delight in our own accomplishments in this activity, it is not unlikely that at times we may envy our skillful patients both their artistic talent and the originality of their imagery.

Along the same lines we may envy their patienthood in art therapy. There have been many occasions when I have seen patients immerse themselves in the art materials I find so inviting. The tender mother-child relationship that art therapy can evoke may arouse longing in the therapist for the child position. The loving acceptance the art therapy patient receives may appear very appealing to those of us who love making art, especially when compared with the harsher reception our art might have received in traditional art training. Envy of our patients, along these and other lines, most often arises from feelings of inadequacy usually rooted in the imperfect nurturing that most of us experienced in early childhood.

Countertransference manifests itself in innumerable ways, but there are a few to which art therapy is especially subject. A defensive maneuver on the part of the therapist may be to set herself above the patient. In art therapy, judgment of patient art is a readily accessible vehicle for such positioning. The art therapist can judge the art, interpret it, use it for assessment and diagnosis. Obviously, these are expectable aspects of the art therapist's work and not simply countertransference maneuvers. The point is that the ambiguity and sometimes mystery of art expression makes it a ready sphere for the enactment of power ploys on the part of the art therapist. In that on most treatment teams the art therapist is the expert on art expression, she is not likely to be challenged by other staff on such judgments.

Communication through art made by the art therapist may also become a countertransference vehicle. For example, a young female student established an art therapy group composed of men with chronic disorders. She made an abstract picture of each man conveying her impressions of him at the group's onset and then at its ending some months later. These pictures were gifts for the men, and the group's dynamics appeared to center around competition for the female art therapist's affection. Without awareness, she was directing the group in such a way as to satisfy her own needs.

The anxiety generated by countertransference issues around the need for control may be manifested in art therapy in an over-structuring of sessions. Rather than being responsive to clients' needs, the art therapist may plan activities in advance without being sufficiently flexible to adapt to immediate conditions and needs. This is especially likely to occur in group art therapy where the sessions may feel more difficult to control. It is sometimes in this way that art therapy becomes gimmicky.

To handle countertransference problems, a responsible art therapist notes her own strong or puzzling feelings in relation to a client or any unexpected behavior on her own part. If she cannot make sense of aspects of her relationship with her client, she seeks professional consultation. Sensitive supervision that focuses on the therapist's self-processes is often helpful (sometimes even less formal interchange with colleagues can be illuminating). Art therapists also have another very potent resource as well—their own art work. Since countertransference, like transference, is an unconscious process, awareness that something is amiss is often difficult to perceive. Consequently, conscientious self-awareness is a necessary first step.

Although art therapists are in the business of encouraging their clients to use art-making for self-understanding, they sometimes fail to avail themselves of its illuminating possibilities for their own self-processing. I have run many workshops in which the task is to examine transference and countertransference relationships through art. By making pictures of one's relationship with a client or a picture of the client, unexpected revelations may surface. Barbara Fish wrote her master's degree thesis on countertransference in art therapy. She systematically used her own art expression to explore her relationships with her patients at her practicum site, a hospital psychiatric unit. Figure 74 was drawn in response to a patient with strong dependency needs who had just lost her boyfriend. Barbara wrote the following about it:

> I became depressed after sessions with the patient and angry that she was
> not stronger. I was unsure why I was so overwhelmed. My intention in

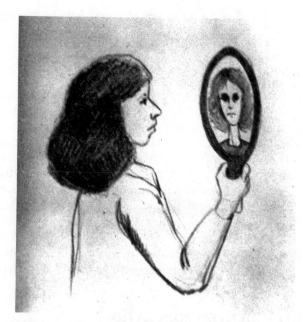

Figure 74. Art therapy student Barbara Fish explored her countertransference to a patient in this self-confrontation.

drawing this picture was to look at my relationship with the patient. Instead, the image I drew represented me looking at myself. The patient's face appeared as the reflection in the mirror instead of my own . . . I saw my own depression in the patient. All the feelings from unsuccessful relationships I have had bubbled to the surface. I projected onto her my own wish for a successful relationship and my rage at men who have not valued me. I saw the depleted nurturer in her face. The face in the mirror reminded me of my mother. My own issues with my mother became clear. The patient was an over-extended giver, caring for children of her own and others. I was reminded of my needs that remained unmet as a child. I was angered that the ability to give is limited. Once I recognized countertransference issues that were stirred by the patient, I could focus on the reality of the therapeutic relationship. This facilitated the progression of her treatment.

The lengths to which Barbara went in her own honest self-exploration are evident. Perhaps in the future it will become a part of an art therapist's regular routine to utilize her own art expression for the illumination of her countertransference issues. At least this process should be used where the art therapist is aware of her own problematic feelings toward clients, patients, or other staff.

Transference Reflections

In addition to the many facets of transference the person of the art therapist and the art therapy activity may evoke is the significant potential the art expression carries for revealing the nature of the transference experience. As such, the substance of art therapy itself (art-making in relationship to another) furnishes its own means of understanding. It not only becomes the meeting place of art therapist and client, but advances the therapy by reflecting images of the therapeutic relationship thereby clarifying dimensions of transference phenomena. These images then become further grist for the therapeutic mill, such as Figure 70.

Grounded in her understanding of the foundation of transference phenomena underpinning the therapeutic relationship, the art therapist encourages its development with greater awareness and sensitivity.

NONINSIGHT ORIENTED POPULATIONS

The therapeutic relationship is of a different nature with noninsight oriented populations than those clients capable of insight. For young children, some retarded people, and those in a state of extreme emotional disturbance, support and understanding are the mainstays of the therapeutic relationship. Santa Claus, Figure 75, would give his first present to me, Figure 76, drawn immediately afterward in pictures made by a six-year-old boy. I did not encourage him to look at his feelings toward me, but rather accepted these depictions as direct expressions of the importance I held for him, his wish to please me, and his affection for me. These pictures were made by the same child who drew the whale, Figure 15. Note the difference in its feeling tone. I tried to help him feel better about himself and be accepting of his feelings through support, often in the form of telling him that it was natural and not "bad" to feel as he did. Much of the therapeutic effort was achieved through my undivided attention and interest and through the offering of art-making, an activity he enjoyed. Art therapy was a "corrective emotional experience" for him, in contrast to his struggles with his mother, father, sister, and teacher.

Figure 77 was made by a disorganized psychotic patient diagnosed acute schizophrenic. He talked constantly while making it, evidencing the intrusion of one idea upon another in the jumbled manner the picture

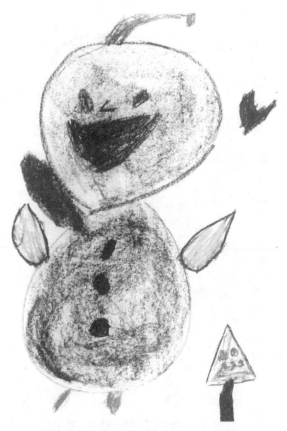

Figure 75. Santa Claus by a six-year-old boy.

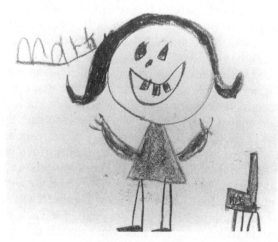

Figure 76. Portrait of the author by a six-year-old boy.

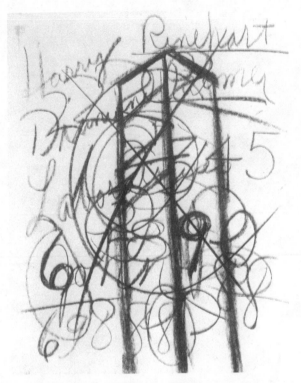

Figure 77. Disorganized drawing by a schizophrenic young man.

illustrates. It was possible only to be present with him, to be supportive where possible, and to provide continuity of the art therapy in anticipation of a less disorganized state when the patient would be more amenable to engagement.

Since I worked with many nonmedicated patients who were diagnosed acute schizophrenic, full-blown manic, and severely depressed, it was not unusual for me to have sessions with people who were difficult to engage. Nevertheless, in almost every case it was possible to gain their cooperation in even the first session. It was necessary to be responsive to these patients without being unduly frightened by their bizarre behavior. For example, one schizophrenic young man threw pastels and kicked the easel. A manic woman slopped paints all over the floor and talked constantly. The depressed elderly man who drew Figure 56 was so withdrawn that he would say nothing about his drawing. For such patients, it is usually impossible to know at the time what the art therapist's interest

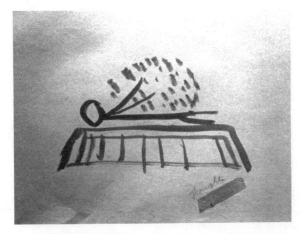

Figure 78. Tears during depression by Rachel, a 48-hour cyclic manic-depressed woman.

means to them during the session. Later indications in almost all cases revealed that my being with them during these difficult times had an important impact. The art produced during these periods of questionable communication offers a picture of the patients' inner state, as shown by the disorganization in Figure 77 and the empty containment in Figure 56.

Rachel, the manic-depressed patient who maintained a 48-hour cycle of mania one day and depression the next (described in Wadeson, 1980, pp. 68–76) provides an example of work with a patient difficult to contact. When depressed, she spoke little, seemed worn out, and sometimes even fell asleep standing before the easel. When manic, she was in perpetual motion, constantly talking, often shouting, moving objects, at times knocking them over, running around (and at times off) the ward in a frenzy. Nursing staff scheduling was planned in advance according to her "high" and "low" days, with an increase in staff for the former. Engagement seemed almost impossible because she was so withdrawn when depressed and so provocative and hyperactive when manic. During depression she seemed unable to speak and during mania unable to listen. There were no in-between periods; she would wake up manic one day and depressed the next. This unrelenting cycle continued for two years.

I began seeing Rachel on depressed days because her manic behavior was so intimidating. My hope was to establish some sort of relationship with her at less stormy times. After a couple of weeks I began scheduling her sessions for one depressed day and one manic day each week. It

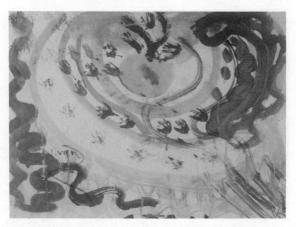

Figure 79. Manic energy seen in a picture painted by Rachel.

became clear that our relationship began to be important to her as she responded to my interest and attention.

In art therapy she became more communicative during depression and less disruptive when manic than she was on the ward. During mania she indicated that she identified with me, seeing us both as artistic women. Although she did not develop much insight during our work together nor improve except to a small degree due to medication administered at a later period, she gained much from the art therapy. She was able to release feelings, even when depressed, and formed one of the few relationships that offered her support during this time. Figure 78, painted in light blue, depicts her depressed feelings as she is showered by her own tears. She dozed off in the midst of painting it while standing at the easel in what appeared to be a successful effort to escape her pain. Figure 79 is representative of her manic high energy. She talked non-stop during its rapid execution, one idea flying into another. At one point she indicated that it was a womb and she titled it "Virgin." Despite her poor attention span when both manic and depressed, Rachel is the patient who sculpted a clay piece of two women seemingly representing herself and me, working on it for several weeks, as described in Chapter 4 under Sculptural Medium. Posing me with my arm around her as she sculpted and describing the affection and care of the one woman for the other, she expressed poignantly the importance of our relationship to her.

Finally a few words about those people who are heavily invested in the art-making process and who may wish to experience their art and demur from "explaining" it. I have encountered this sort of situation in workshops rather than in ongoing treatment. In the latter an expectation of self-exploration is developed. I think the art therapist's position once again is that of support and interest plus acknowledgment of the importance of the art to its creator. It is best not to be invasive or intrusive. Where the artwork is invested with much importance for these individuals, they are likely to reflect on it further after the session and to benefit from it in ways not easily verbalized. When working with those who take their art seriously, simply being with them and helping to incubate the sometimes mysterious process of image development is a very significant and personal sort of sharing. Patience is necessary as images evolve and eventually tell their own story.

MAKING ART WITH CLIENTS

A further way to relate to clients through art is by making art with them. Some art therapists do so as a regular practice. I seldom do because: (1) I want to give my full attention to the client; (2) I don't want my art expressions to be a distraction from the client's work; (3) I don't want to take precious therapy time to process my art; and (4) I am more experienced in art than most clients, so my art may be intimidating or may provide a model of what they "should" do.

Nevertheless, there are occasions where I have found my own art a powerful and useful means of communication in art therapy. A new group was spending several hours outside meditating and sketching, each one working alone. My thoughts were primarily of them, so I sketched them, Figure 80. It was a way of beginning to know them and communicating with them. The drawings are tentative and realistic as I had not seen these people before and my impressions were primarily visual.

Figure 81, on the other hand, is a much bolder representation of myself. Another out-patient group, this time one well-seasoned, was sharing experiences of being disoriented. I suggested making pictures of these experiences. I felt it important to participate, to share that I too had had such experiences. I drew myself in the shower after having taken medication. I had no sense of time and thought I had been there forever and never would come out. The black surrounding represents my spatial disorientation as well. When I closed my eyes, despite the water sprinkling my skin, I did not know where I was. As this group was composed of all women, my nakedness here is self-disclosure rather than sexual provocativeness. Figure 81 is far more expressive than Figure 80.

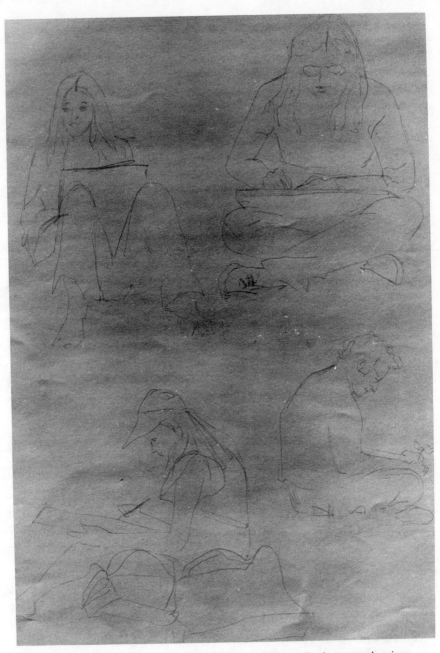

Figure 80. The author's sketches of group members while they were drawing.

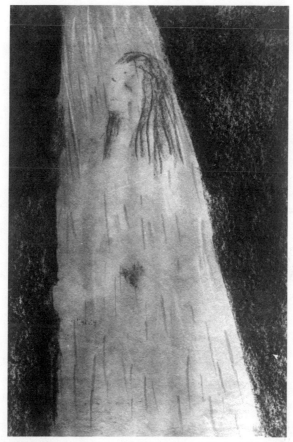

Figure 81. The author's self-representation of being disoriented.

Another well-seasoned out-patient group, also one composed of all women, was exploring the archetype of the wicked witch, at first fearing her and then identifying with her. Once again, I thought it important to join them in this experience as a woman who also struggles with conflicts over my own power including my possibilities for evil. It was with great relish that I drew the evil witch in Figure 82. My lack of inhibition in making her as menacing as I could was very freeing to some of the others. These latter two examples illustrate how the art therapist may utilize the art for therapist transparency as well as for joining with clients.

I want to emphasize that the occasions for my own art expression in art

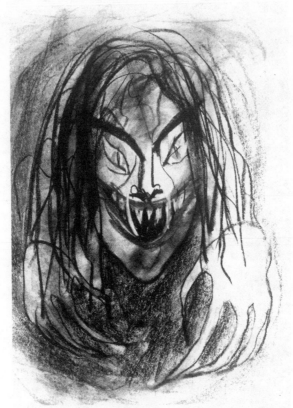

Figure 82. The author's drawing of a wicked witch.

therapy sessions are highly selective. Because it is art-making time and this is an activity the art therapist enjoys are not sufficient reasons for an art therapist to make art with clients. I believe the art therapist should work with self-awareness and understand the important ramifications of how she participates with clients. Generally what I am trying to convey is that art therapy is not a time and place where we make art, but rather an occasion for therapy, for dealing with the client's issues through art.

Art-Making Together

Although the art therapist does not work on the client's art, there may be occasions where they create a piece together. In these instances the art

therapist remains sensitive to the client's leads and needs. One oc
where I created a picture with a patient was with a middle-aged man who
had just made a very serious suicide attempt. He would neither talk nor
make art. With the suggestion that we make a picture together, he was
willing to enter in. The nonverbal communication we achieved as we
worked in turn, each one adding something to what the other had drawn,
allowed for a special sort of togetherness that seemed important to this
patient at this moment.

A different sort of example stands out in my memory from my early
days in art therapy. I was experiencing a strain in the relationship with my
art therapy supervisor at that time so we decided to do a picture together.
We started with the "scribble technique" in which a picture is developed
from a random scribble made with eyes closed. It evolved into a fish with
a little girl lying on its back, her feet up in the air and her eyes closed. The
fish appeared to be taking her for a ride. I felt that the little girl was me and
that I was closing my eyes to much of what was going on as I rode
passively on the back of my supervisor. It seemed time for me to wake up
and swim for myself. We were able to take a look at the picture we had
created together as a reflection of the relationship we had created together.

Sequence drawings in which the client and therapist alternate drawing
panels to tell a story are often useful in work with children. The child
begins the sequence, and the art therapist responds. In this way, the art
therapist can suggest possible alternatives. Figure 83 is an example.
Tommy was an angry, sometimes withdrawn 10-year-old. He related defi-
antly and had no friends. Most of his drawings depicted his active fantasy
life in which mechanical beings and monsters destroyed people and fought
each other. Tommy began a sequence drawing with one of his favorites,
"Mighty Machine Man." I responded in the second panel with a boy and
a dog approaching in a friendly way. In the third panel, Tommy's "Mighty
Machine Man" laughs as he destroys them. I realized that I needed to
enter Tommy's world, rather than to try to introduce people into it. In the
fourth panel, I gave his mechanical monster a mother who presents him
with a birthday cake saying, "Happy birthday, Mighty." Her name is
"Mother Machine." I tried to draw a warm feminine version of his Machine Man. To my surprise, in the next panel Tommy showed his Machine
Man as vulnerable with a stomach ache from eating the whole cake,
"candles and all." For the final panel, I drew Mother Machine taking care
of him, tucking him into bed and saying, "Sleep well, Mighty. Pleasant
dreams." Tommy seemed pleased and worked peacefully on a drawing of
a horse until the end of the session.

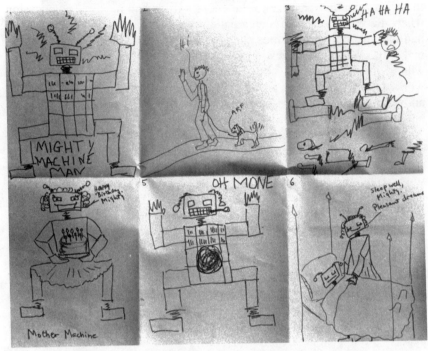

Figure 83. A sequence drawing made by the art therapist and a child.

CONCLUSION

The skill and creativity of the art therapist are nowhere more important than in how she relates to her clients and patients through and around their art expressions. This is the heart of art therapy requiring her full presence and awareness of self, client, art, and life. With training and experience, with the accumulation of lessons learned from many clients, the art therapist continuously refines her sensitivity in an ongoing development that proceeds throughout all her professional life.

Finally, it is important to realize that it is not possible to work in the complex and subtle realms of psychotherapy without ever making a mistake. There may be times when there is misunderstanding, misinterpretation, some minor exploitation. If art therapists are generally and genuinely conscientious, these missteps will not be unduly damaging and the client will benefit from the balance of the positive work. The most any clinician can do is to try to develop awareness of her own motives and the consequences of her own interventions to the fullest degree she can. This is an ongoing process. It not only strengthens her own integrity, but it also serves as a model for clients in their learning not to fool themselves and to be responsible to themselves and to others.

For further discussion of developing the therapeutic relationship, see Wadeson (1980, Chapter 6). Sources outside art therapy that I have found helpful in their discussions of the therapeutic relationship are:

Bruch, H. *Learning Psychotherapy*, 1974

Kopp, S. *If You Meet the Buddha on the Road, Kill Him*, 1972

Guggenbuhl-Craig, A.: *Power in the Helping Professions*, 1971

Reik, T. *Listening With the Third Ear*, 1949

Yalom, I. *The Theory and Practice of Group Psychotherapy*, 1975

Yalom, I. & Elkins, G. *Every Day Gets a Little Closer*, 1974

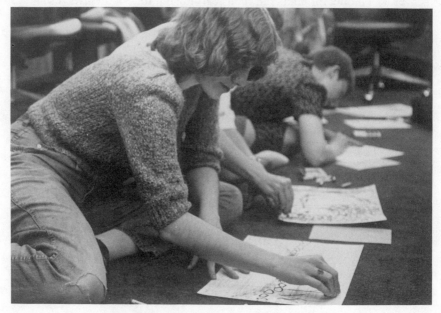

Figure 84. Terry Reimer drawing in a group.

CHAPTER 6

Group Art Therapy

Although my previous book (*Art Psychotherapy*, 1980) contains a chapter on group art therapy, I want to give it further discussion in this volume because it is such a prominent part of most art therapists' work and there is minimal material in the literature addressing this important area.

Many treatment facilities can justify employment of an art therapist only if she sees many individuals. This, of course, is best accomplished in groups. The opportunity for large numbers to experience art therapy is certainly not the prime advantage of group art therapy nor its most significant *raison d'etre*. In fact, viewed from this factory-like orientation, it is likely little more than watered down individual art therapy. Recently an art therapist in her first job told me that the school for emotionally disturbed children where she works requires her to see 20 adolescents together in a group, despite her protestations. What the administrators must have in mind is an activity period to give the adolescents something to do, rather than anything that could be considered therapy.

In addition to an institution's making unreasonable demands of group art therapy, there may be shortcomings on the art therapist's part as well. To maximize group art therapy's fullest potential, the art therapist must be well-versed in understanding and operating among the complex forces of group dynamics. In addition, she needs to know how art expression can be best utilized in this sort of force field. Unfortunately, little has been published in the latter area. Although there are many books and articles on group dynamics and group therapy, these essential requirements for adequate preparation of an art therapist may be neglected in training. This chapter provides an effort to add to the meager body of knowledge on group art therapy.

There are two possible directions group art therapy may take. One is built upon the dynamic approach formulated for group therapy. The other is based on the communal sharing of image-making and image-understanding. There is overlap between the two approaches, but they will be discussed here separately for purposes of clarification. Naturally there is variety within the different approaches as well, determined by population, setting, and so forth. Of particular influence is the factor of time. Goals must be limited and methods considerably modified in short-term treatment as will be discussed later. Another significant consideration is the functional abilities of the group members, also considered in this chapter.

GROUP DYNAMICS APPROACH

A leading articulator of group therapy and practice is Irvin Yalom (*The Theory and Practice of Group Therapy*, 1975). He describes group therapy as a form of treatment based on the interpersonal model of human development. This is a concept postulated most explicitly by Harry Stack Sullivan (1940, 1953) stressing the importance of relationships with significant other human beings in shaping the development of the growing child. In a quest for security the child maximizes those traits that meet with approval and squelches those that are disapproved until the sense of self becomes made up of perceived appraisals by others. Consequently, Sullivan conceived of therapy as directed toward the processes between people. Based on this view of human development, group therapy is interpersonally based in both its goals and its means. It is a suitable mode of treatment, therefore, for objectives such as dealing with loneliness, problems in intimacy, lack of confidence in dealing with others, and many other interpersonal problems.

The means of therapy are interpersonal as well, in that each group member creates his or her own social microcosm within the group, displaying the unique interpersonal difficulties that have led to treatment. Group therapy of this kind tends to be relatively ahistorical as the therapist helps to keep the focus on the here-and-now. Through self-observation and feedback from others in the group, members come to appreciate the nature of their behavior and its impact on others; to contemplate and risk change; to gain experience of change and feedback on it in the group; and eventually to bring change to their lives outside the group. These changes move in the direction of more satisfactory interpersonal relationships which then enhance self-esteem.

In group therapy an essential component of a well-functioning group is the development of trust. This is a condition that takes time. As trust grows, the group is likely to become more cohesive, that is, more meaningful to its members. Increased cohesiveness encourages further possibilities for risk and change and subsequently more trust in an evolving spiral of therapeutic work at greater depth and with increasing positive growth of individual members. Naturally, the course is seldom smooth, and there are often set-backs along the way.

With this very brief overview of the premises of group therapy, let us take a look at what happens in group art therapy. In group art therapy, trust and cohesiveness take on a further dimension. The world of images is a private one. Not only that, self-revelation in art may be more difficult to control than in verbal communication. (See Wadeson, 1980, p. 9.) Further, art-making may entail performance fear as discussed in Chapter 3. For all these reasons group members may feel at greater risk and need more trust for this sort of sharing of private, not easily controlled, imagery. There is a reciprocal relationship between risk and trust. A risk that has proved worth taking usually increases trust. Thus, having risked exposure of a vulnerable image, a group member usually feels more trusting of the group and the total group develops an atmosphere of greater trust. Reciprocally again, such trust encourages the likelihood that other risky images will be shared, both by the person who has already risked and by the others who have witnessed the beneficial outcome of the risk.

The producing and sharing of images within a group lead to some significant results. A very special intimacy develops as a consequence of the sort of risk-taking and trust-building described above. Group members come to know one another in a new way, a way in which individuals in our society seldom know one another, including those in verbal therapy groups. Visual languages are developed, expressed, and shared. The dimension of imagistic conceptualization and expression is exposed and communicated. Through this sharing, those in an art therapy group come to know one another's imagistic symbols, styles, themes, and to be known by the others for the characteristics of their own visual expression.

Some of the processes that occur are difficult to discuss because they are not experienced verbally and in some cases there are not words adequate to describe them. The process of art-making in the company of others, particularly where indepth ongoing relationships develop, is not easy to explain. Often there is a feeling of community, even when all work is in silence. It's quite a different experience from making art in solitude. The presence of the others and their participation in the same activity creates an ambiance. Usually it is an experience of support for the work and stimulation of ideas, energy, and creativity. Creating, (i.e., making something) is an enlivening activity. Beyond the physical activation that occurs, the creative activation heightens individual and group energy. Such activation at times contrasts with the relative passivity of a purely verbal group where members are usually planted in stationary chairs and may create little in their verbalization.

Participation and competition are factors in any group. In an art therapy group they take on a different cast. In verbal groups some people may participate more than others and issues of a particular member may dominate one or more sessions. In art therapy, usually everyone produces an art object or if not becomes a focus of attention for abstaining. It is rare that any art expression would be neglected by the group. Usually, each art expression arouses too much curiosity to be side-stepped. The spatial nature of art, as opposed to the temporal nature of verbal expression, puts each member's imagery before the others; each member presents himself or herself, even those who are most withdrawn. In this way, all become a part of the group focus. Whereas in verbal therapy a withdrawn or resistant group member may need to be invited or even prodded to enter the discussion, in art therapy usually all are "in," having communicated to the others in visual expression even before speaking.

Another part of the group art therapy process that is difficult to reduce to words is the impact of visual communication. Although there is usually discussion of the art productions, the initial message they give is imagistic. This message is received by other group members and it impacts on them whether they can describe their reactions or not. The same can be said for the reactions to one's own art expression, both the experience of making it and the viewing of it as it develops and upon completion. Words often fail to convey the entire experience. This is an understandable condition. If words were sufficient, the art experience would be unnecessary. It is because art taps into reservoirs of being that are not necessarily verbally articulatable that it is of significant communicative import. Therefore, the impact of one's art expression on oneself and the others as well as receiving the impact from others' art becomes a part of each individual's experience and a significant dimension of the life of the group as a whole.

Competition for attention, approval, special status, jockeying for position or to achieve impact—the sibling rivalry that characterizes early relationships in group therapy—also play a part in the dynamics of group art therapy. Added to this is the element of art competition. In a well-working group, this factor usually dissipates after the initial phase, but early on it may have a considerable influence. Heightening performance fear may be odious comparisons with artistic skills, imagination, and originality of other group members. This added dimension may reshuffle group roles and power structure that otherwise might develop around other sorts of skills, such as verbal articulateness, seductiveness, interpersonal competencies, and so forth. An extreme example would be a withdrawn individual who draws compelling pictures, such as the silent

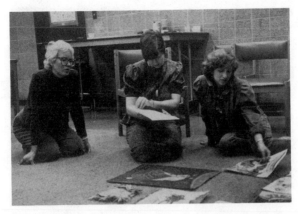

Figure 85. Deborah Behnke-Marthaler, Susan Werler, and Diane Evans discussing their art expressions.

adolescent who drew Figure 13. The group pulled him out of his shell with their interest in his imagery.

The primary benefit of group art therapy is the sharing of images with others. Although the very act of creating images is often a powerful experience, this activity may be obtained through individual art therapy. The group becomes the world in microcosm and it is upon this sea that the images are set to sail. Where the winds will take them is part of the adventure.

But to what ends is this journey directed? As stated previously, the objectives are interpersonal. My first art therapy experience was over two decades ago with two adolescent groups at the NIH. The major writings on group therapy had yet to be written. Nevertheless, my observations led me to note that the groups' most significant foci were "common experiences" and "feelings about each other" (Sinrod, 1964). It was not until many years later when I was teaching group therapy that I found confirmation in Yalom's articulation of "universality" and the "here-and-now social microcosm" (Yalom, 1975). It's surprising to me that my naive observations of what was most consequential at a time when I had received no training are the same as I hold now, several graduate degrees and many groups later.

People who come to therapy usually consider their problems unique and feel isolated in bearing troubles they believe no one else encounters. In some instances the isolation is so pervasive that the individual assumes that no one else can understand. The feeling about the self may be so

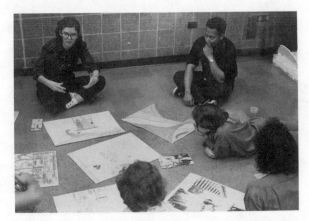

Figure 86. Typically informal processing of a group's drawings.

deprecating that the individual assumes that no one else would even want
to understand. To those who feel worthless, it may come as a startling
revelation to discover that others feel that way too.

Sharing of images, whether around specific problems or pervasive feelings, can be a dramatic revelation of commonality. In contrast to a statement such as "I've felt that way too" or "I've had that experience also,"
an art representation *shows* the feeling or experience. It is usually spontaneous and unbidden and often has an emotional impact. Thus, the group
member comes to feel a part of a group in which there are understanding
individuals who perhaps share some specific problems, but who certainly
experience universal concerns, such as making life meaningful, intimacy
and separateness from others, loss, anger, disappointment, and eventually the transitory quality of life.

In this atmosphere of support and understanding, one can begin to
examine one's behavior in terms of how it impacts on others and to
change, redefine one's sense of self, and establish more satisfactory relationships. Once again, imagistic expression is a natural and impactful
vehicle for this sort of discovery.

The here-and-now focus on the developing social microcosm in the art
therapy group is one of its most powerful forces for change. As in verbal
group therapy, one of the therapist's major tasks is process illumination
(Yalom, 1975). Illumination of process includes both individual interactions as well as mass group commentary directed toward the culture of the
group as a whole. For example, an individual process illumination might
be: "Jack, it looks as though your constant talking is an effort to deal with

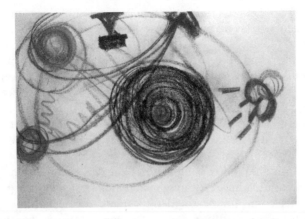

Figure 87. Therapist as large sun around which group members orbit.

your anxiety over your pass to go home.'' An example of a mass group commentary would be: ''It appears that the group is avoiding doing its work in letting Jack talk nonstop through the whole session.''

In group art therapy, process may become illuminated through images as well as words and additionally through reflection on the images. Individual feedback may be eloquently given as group members make pictures of one another. The development of the group as a whole may be seen in each member's view of the group at a particular time (Figure 87) or an issue facing the group presented in art expression. Reflection on the individual images produced may reveal a group theme or mood by observing content and affect respectively. Group projects, such as murals, may reveal interactive processes as well as group themes. Often times the art is so dramatically revealing that the sort of therapist process illumination needed in verbal group therapy only underscores what is already evident to the group as displayed in the art. On the other hand, when group processes are not so evident, the art may serve as a useful reference point for the therapist's commentary.

An important aspect of the utilization of art in group therapy is its important place not only in reflecting group process, as previously described, but in its advancing group process. This advancement occurs simultaneously with the sort of reflection that group images provide. For example, when group members draw pictures of the group, awareness becomes magnified. Each person has shared his or her view; common constellations are identified; different perceptions are recognized; feelings about the group are communicated; each member has access to the position he or she holds in every member's conception of the group. Usually, there has been risk in divulging these perceptions. All this information and sharing of feeling adds substantially to the growth of the group. As a result, the group ends the session in a far different place from where it began. The visual images of the group not only displayed its reflection in the eyes of each group member but each member's visual expression and apprehension of the others' images moved the group process in the direction of greater awareness, understanding, and usually closeness, cohesiveness, and trust. The experience is likely to be a holistic one. Although each member's depiction may be viewed individually, taken together all the images form a complex composite of the life of the group.

There is a paradox here. Although each member enters the group as an individual, has come for personal treatment, and leaves the group for personal reasons (hopefully when his or her treatment has been completed), at the same time his or her individual odyssey in the group is part of the total group experience and impacts on all other members. Thus the group therapist and group art therapist must maintain a double vision: one that focuses on each individual member's progress as well as a vision of the development of the group as an embracing culture shaped by and shaping each member. The art expressions often add clarity to this dual focus.

Having discussed group art therapy in general terms, let's take a look at the sort of material that is likely to be explored in this process. Obviously, there are infinite possibilities, many of which are determined by the nature of the group. Some groups are formed for specific purposes, such as a mothers' group for learning disabled children. The group's goal might be to help the mothers deal with their children more effectively and as such would focus on their relationships with the children and others involved with the children. For problems with self-esteem, marital therapy, and so forth, they would likely be referred elsewhere or seen individually by the therapist.

Several specialized groups I conducted were composed of alcoholics being treated in an alcohol abuse program. The clients were mostly court-referred and participated in 10 sessions. The groups were often large with changing compositions as people entered and left the program. As a result, the focus remained pretty much the same: what part alcohol consumption played in their lives. Figures 88 and 89 are two experiences shared with the group.

Ongoing groups that have a more general focus run the gamut of life experience. At the heart of much of the material, however, is self-concept. Figure 52 is an example from such a group.

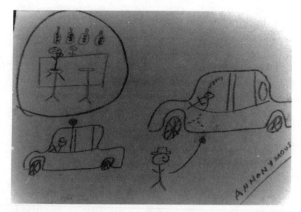

Figure 88. The part alcohol consumption played in his life by a man arrested for drunk driving, drawn in an alcohol abuse treatment group.

An early task of most therapy groups is dealing with authority. In contrast to individual therapy, the group therapy member does not have the therapist all to oneself. The competitive feelings for approval, attention, power as mediated by the therapist, are significant interpersonal learning experiences. The transference phenomena evoked have important repercussions for dealing with authority in group situations through-

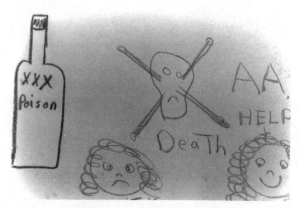

Figure 89. A woman's experience of her alcoholism drawn in an alcohol abuse treatment group.

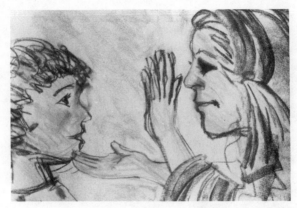

Figure 90. A young woman's drawing of her relationship to the group leader, right.

out one's life. Art expression provides a compelling picture of the situation. Figure 90 is an example showing me on the right and the young woman who drew it on the left. She wrote the following about it:

> In my relationship to Harriet personally I felt both an invitation to be open and at other times an abrupt coolness. The drawing is about all the ambivalence. Harriet is beckoning to me with one hand and stopping me with the other. I am anxious about how we will get along. When I shared the drawing

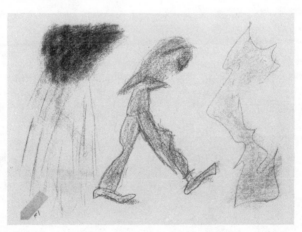

Figure 91. A hospitalized adolescent portrayed a frightening group member walking from a storm toward a fire.

in the group, I was scared of how Harriet might react. I was pleased that I found the courage to share some negative feelings about her. Her accepting response was helpful in defusing the conflict I felt.

Other important issues include the commonality of experiences as mentioned above (universality). The images produced by the alcoholic groups (Figures 88 and 89) are instances where I deliberately suggested topics of common experience. In ongoing groups of longer duration and greater stability of membership, the focus of a common experience may develop spontaneously.

Peer relationships become important as illustrated in Figure 91. In a group of hospitalized adolescents, one member experienced another in the group as frightening due to his sudden, explosive, angry outbursts. Spontaneously, she communicated her view of him to the group in a depiction of him emerging from a storm to enter fire.

SHORT-TERM GROUPS

Many art therapists work on psychiatric units where patients are hospital- ized for only a few weeks and the ward population changes daily. The trust and cohesion that are important components of long-term groups are impossible to attain in short-term groups due both to the instability of the population and the greater disturbance and poorer functioning of the pa- tients. Many art therapists feel quite frustrated by these conditions. Sel- dom is there opportunity to build a therapeutic alliance and to be a part of the human growth that can be so gratifying in long-term work.

Yalom (1983) states that the goal of short-term, in-patient group ther- apy is to prepare patients to continue therapy after discharge. Frankly, I question whether under the usual difficult circumstances of short-term, in-patient group therapy such a goal is realistic. It seems to me that a more relevant goal would be sharing feelings about hospitalization and the con- ditions of the particular facility. With patients who are too disturbed to communicate with one another or to share attention, group therapy is probably not worth the effort. In such cases the art therapist is better advised to schedule frequent individual sessions.

Where group art therapy appears to be feasible and beneficial, the circumstances require a more structured approach than in the more stable long-term group. The following section discusses structure of various kinds of art therapy groups. After an exposition of the many factors involved in establishing a group, structured group art therapy activities, including those appropriate for short-term work, will be presented.

STRUCTURE

As discussed in Chapter 2, the physical arrangement of the art therapy room and the kinds of art materials used are an important influence. Whereas it is possible to be flexible in scheduling individual art therapy sessions as to both time and place, group art therapy almost always necessitates a consistent meeting time and place. On a hospital unit an art therapy room that is on the ward obviates the sometimes difficult task of escorting a group of disturbed patients from one part of the hospital to another.

More significant, however, is the cooperation of the rest of the staff in an institutional setting in their support of group art therapy (see Chapter 11). For example, when I was conducting a group composed of withdrawn and lethargic psychotic depressives, actively suicidal individuals, and full-blown manics, it was seldom possible to begin on time. I had to round up the patients, even though the meeting room was on the ward, and received little cooperation from staff who were busy giving medications and taking care of other responsibilities. After negotiation, however, we were able to plan the schedule so that medications were completed and staff were available to summon stragglers to the session.

Screening and Composition

In short-term treatment, it is likely that all admissions would participate in art therapy. On the other hand, as previously mentioned, many groups might be formed for particular purposes with particular populations (such as mothers of learning disabled children). In long-term work, however, the group therapist is something of a match-maker, trying to fit into the group people who will work well together. The prime criterion for such selection is functional level. And in fact, many hospital psychiatric units are organized around low and high level functional groups. (See Yalom, 1983, for a detailed discussion of "level" group therapy.) Often a group can move only as fast as its slowest member, and others may lose interest when they are otherwise ready to move ahead. A dramatic example of discordant functioning I experienced occurred when I was conducting group therapy for a psychologist in private practice. The group was composed of well-functioning professionals who met in an office at the psychologist's home. We had agreed that I would screen anyone she wanted to refer to the group. Contrary to our agreement, she admitted a woman I had not screened. After the woman's first session, I told the psychologist I thought the new member was psychotic, needed individual treatment (in the group she had demanded a great deal of individual attention), and was not ready for the group. The psychologist insisted that she remain, and as it was clear she had no intention of living up to our agreements, I resigned. A few weeks later I learned that the psychologist removed the woman from the group after she drove her car through the bay window of the office!

Another factor group therapists should consider in composition is deviancy. Diversity is fine in age, sex, ethnicity, socio-economic status, and so forth. But one member who is a group deviant in any of these areas is likely to remain singled out throughout the group's life. One group I conducted that had been organized by the same psychologist was composed of all women except for one man. He remained "special" in the group, sometimes being asked to present "the male point of view." As he had grown up as the "special" only son among three sisters, this situation provided little in the way of a corrective emotional experience for him.

Obviously group members do not enter the group as perfect candidates. If they were, they probably would not need therapy. Therefore, many may be closed, defensive, withdrawn, dominating, and so forth. These are not reasons for exclusion, but rather interpersonal stances that are grist for the group mill.

In group art therapy, occasionally art experience may be a screening factor as well. For example, I have conducted several groups composed of art therapists and art therapy students. Naturally they were all experienced and comfortable with art expression. Although others entered these groups, an individual with little art experience who was uncomfortable in art expression would have felt disadvantaged.

Generally, the optimal size for a therapy group is five to 10. In art therapy it is even more important than in a verbal group that the size not grow too large. It's a matter of time: Making art takes time and reflecting on each art expression takes time. It's frustrating to have to postpone discussion of some of the art until the next session. Much is lost in the way of immediate feelings and reactions.

Time Factors

One and a half to two hours is the usual length of ongoing sessions. It's difficult to discuss all the art in less time, and people tend to run out of steam after about two hours. If the group is composed of disturbed individuals, one hour or even less might be the extent of attention span. Prolonged sessions, such as all day or weekend workshops, will be discussed separately.

To establish continuity, a therapy group should meet at least weekly. In short-term settings where patients are discharged rapidly and sometimes suddenly, more frequent sessions are advisable because patients may remain in the group only two or three weeks. Yalom (1983) suggests daily meetings if possible.

An art therapy group may be open-ended with people entering and leaving according to their own timetables for beginning and ending treatment. Or a group may be time-limited, meeting for a designated number of sessions. Group members may attend voluntarily, by professional referral, or as a part of a required program. Decisions about these matters should be made purposefully, rather than randomly, depending on goals and conditions of work. Regardless, a commitment on the part of the art therapist and group members is necessary for effective work.

Cotherapy

Two art therapists may conduct a group together, but more often when there is cotherapy in an art therapy group the art therapist is paired with another mental health professional. This sort of cotherapy relationship provides an excellent opportunity for other team members to learn firsthand just what art therapy entails and what it can provide. Under these circumstances, usually the art therapist takes the lead in encouraging the art, in designing any structured activities that are used, and in processing the art. The cotherapist may lead in areas of his/her expertise. For example, when I was asked to help family therapists Lyman Wynne and Carl Whitaker in the study of a family, I accompanied Lyman to a home visit where he led the interview, and I played an auxiliary role when he and Carl conducted a televised interview. On the other hand, when Lyman and I conducted an art therapy session with the family, I designed the tasks, selected the art materials, and led the family discussion of their products.

In ongoing work, cotherapy can be almost as complicated and involving as a marriage. A cotherapist offers an additional vantage point and understanding, as well as a partner who can provide support and responsibility for the tasks of group leadership. Sometimes group experience can become so intense that it helps to be able to sit back and rest for a short time and leave the driving to your cotherapist. Cotherapists can take on different roles in the group. One can focus on the group as a whole while the other is being alert to individual reactions. With two therapists, transference projections may be diluted.

A male/female cotherapy team stimulates the possibility of constituting the family constellation and projections can be readily examined. For example, in a couples group I led with a male psychiatrist, some members were confronted with their habitual stereotypes. My cotherapist was male with higher credentials (I did not have a Ph.D. at the time), and we met in his offices. Yet I was more active in the group taking on a greater proportion of the leadership since he had no prior group experience. This was confounding to some of the group members—they expected that the male doctor would lead. Eventually it surfaced that one of the members had assumed that we were lovers (we weren't). We worked well together and obviously had a warm relationship. This client's experience led her to believe that warmth between a man and woman occurred only in a sexual relationship. Further, she had fantasized that the psychiatrist was married and I was divorced (we were both divorced). She was confronted with still another stereotype about love, marriage, and sex roles in our society.

Competition, misunderstandings, working at cross-purposes, unmet expectations, and poor communication can beleaguer a cotherapy relationship. These are some of the factors that make working with a partner difficult. Cotherapy takes time and effort. Cotherapists model the negotiations and clarifications that are necessary for any close ongoing relationship. Superficial politeness where there are underlying difficulties gives clients mixed messages about the very areas of interpersonal relationships that the group is established to effect.

In art therapy groups there is the additional task of educating the nonart therapist to the considerations necessary in group art therapy so that the two do not operate at odds.

Preparation

If possible, the art therapist (and her cotherapist if she has one) should meet with prospective group members individually prior to their entrance into the group. There are three reasons for this: (1) to screen the individual to determine his appropriateness for the group and the group's appropriateness for him; (2) to prepare him for the group by letting him know what is expected of him, including some information about art therapy and how the group operates in terms of openness, confidentiality, and goals; and (3) to establish contact with him so that when he enters a group of strangers, at least he knows the therapist(s) a bit.

Most groups have ground rules established by the therapist. They usually include attendance, punctuality, encouragement of openness and honesty, a disregard for certain social conventions of politeness, and a prohibition of physical violence. Art therapy groups might also encourage free use of the materials so long as they are properly cleaned up and put away. It is useful to stress that the purpose is self-expression rather than artistic accomplishment. I also establish a framework for commenting on other members' art, to the effect that comments about others' art are statements about the person who has made them, rather than definitive analyses of another. All of this is a new experience for the group art therapy members, so the art therapist must often refer to the group rules in the initial sessions in building the group culture. For example, if a member "analyzes" another's picture, the art therapist might turn it back to him and ask him how the picture makes him feel.

Structured Activities

Short-term art therapy groups generally require more structured art activities. There is not time to allow the natural unfolding and development of each individual's visual language. Therefore, if the art therapist determines that a useful focus would be reaction to hospitalization, she might suggest that each group member make a picture of how it feels to be in the hospital. In the discussion of the pictures, she would be active in drawing connections among the pictures and trying to involve all the participants in discussion. Other common feelings and experiences might be addressed through the art as well, such as structured tasks to explore plans after discharge, family relationships, and so forth. The amount of time for art-making and discussion would be determined by the art therapist on the basis of her perception of the needs of the group. If there are new members attending the session, she would try to introduce them and integrate them to help them feel less uncomfortable.

In a new group, either long or short-term, it is sometimes easier for people to relate to one other person initially than to the group as a whole. The art therapist, therefore, may ask people to pair up to discuss their art. Pairing may be applied to artwork as well. Making a picture together can be too threatening initially but when people are ready, it is an excellent way for them to observe their own patterns of leadership, cooperation, competition, territoriality, and so forth. Usually the shared fantasy and creativity go a long way in establishing a bond between the two.

Murals are an excellent way to help develop group cohesiveness (Figure 92). The group may select a theme or group symbol, or one may arise

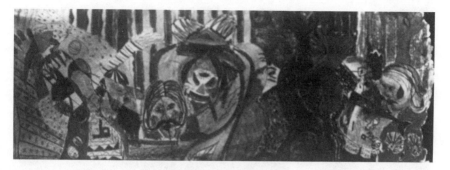

Figure 92. A group mural.

spontaneously. Sometimes unplanned group murals are chaotic but fun nevertheless. Reflecting on them often provides much information about group patterning, such as leadership, connectedness versus separateness, territoriality, competition, and so forth.

A ground-breaker for new groups with much performance fear and a need to connect with one another is the round robin. Each person works on a picture for a short time (two or three minutes). The art therapist calls "time" or "switch" and each person passes his/her picture to the person to the right (or left). The process continues until each person has worked on every picture and each picture has gone around the circle and returned to its originator. By that time, the initial drawing is often unrecognizable. There is usually humor and curiosity about who did what. Feelings can be examined and reactions explored. In one round robin a woman covered a bird with a black grid because the picture was too "pretty and sweet." Another woman who worked on it subsequently obliterated the grid and asserted the bird, coloring it more brilliantly because she wanted it to be "free," Figure 93. Often the various pictures from one round robin contain different moods and themes. These may be explored in terms of what they say about the group. Performance fear is avoided because each picture is made by all group members, and each one's contribution may be unrecognizable.

As mentioned earlier in this chapter, pictures of the group and its members are especially revealing and involving. They provide one of the best ways for group participants to give one another feedback. As a result, group cohesiveness usually advances.

Also mentioned earlier is the emerging theme that might arise in the group's work. Examples of this process as well as group depictions and

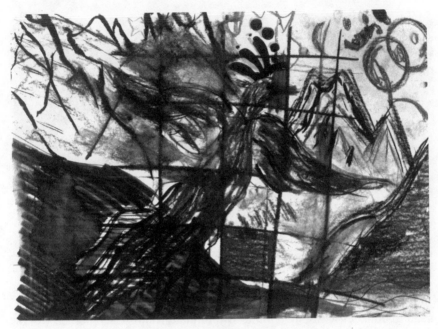

Figure 93. A group "round robin" picture.

feelings about the leader and others in the group may be found in Wadeson, *Art Psychotherapy,* 1980, Chapter 19.

The most significant question regarding structured art activities (including guided imagery) is not what to use, but whether and when one
should use them at all. Recently I sat in on a class of about 20 art therapists and a few art therapy students. The group went "round" three
times, each telling of an art therapy technique he or she used. In a short
time, we had heard about 60 techniques. Most people took notes. The
student next to me titled hers, "Recipes for Art Therapy."

Art therapy isn't a piece of cake. An art therapist isn't there to provide
projects. If she trusts the power of imagery and the healing forces within
her client, she will allow her groups to flow naturally and organically. She
will trust that matters that need to be dealt with will surface in the imagery. And she will trust herself to be sensitive to their emergence so that
she can foster their exploration and encourage the growth potential of the
art therapy group and its individual members. A cutesy project may be
fun and rewarding to its maker, but it hardly develops insight. Elaborate
projects that are conceived and guided by the art therapist do not gener-

ally contribute to the creativity discussed in the next section of this chapter. It is in this regard that an art therapist must be a therapist first and foremost, not an art teacher or recreation therapist. For the most part, therefore, except in specially focused groups, the art activities will grow organically out of each group's unique development.

COMMUNAL SHARING OF IMAGE-MAKING

In communal sharing of image making the emphasis is on the development of images more than the insight derived from them. In this respect it is akin to "art as therapy," but unlike the latter, there is also an emphasis on the shared experience. To describe this process is very difficult because it does not readily lend itself to words.

Such groups seldom adhere to a traditional art therapy format. More often they are of a workshop nature, lasting a half-day, full day, weekend, week, or may be ongoing over months, meeting periodically. The longer session allows for meditation, incubation, creating, and sharing. Groups are usually composed of people committed to art-making who for one reason or another want to share that process with a group. Such a group differs from an art class in that although there is a strong investment in the art process and creativity, the goal is not art excellence, but rather a personal "in-touchness" with oneself and a sharing of the experience. The "Pursuit of the Image" workshops I have conducted (Chapter 12) fall into this category.

The role of the art therapist in these groups differs from that in the "group dynamics approach." She may be a facilitator, as I was in "Pursuit of the Image" workshops, setting structure and giving direction. Usually she also participates as a group member as well, creating her own art. Processing the art and sharing the experience becomes an individual responsibility with little prompting by the art therapist other than her structuring the group so that there is opportunity for such sharing. Seldom does she ask probing questions, for example.

Because sessions are often lengthier, more elaborate projects may be developed. Figures 94 and 95 are masks made in one such group. Group members paired up to apply plaster gauze to one another's faces so that each mask began as a mold of one's face (Figures 96 and 97). There was sharing of the feelings involved, such as being unable to talk, having one's eyes covered, the gentleness of the applier's touch.

Another group made a series of tissue paper collages, letting each one

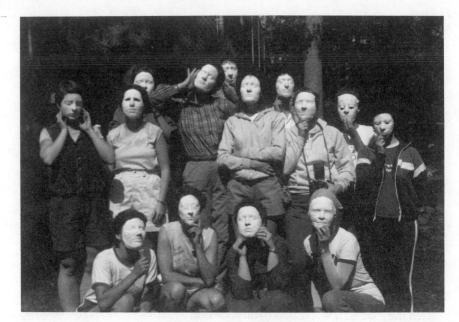

Figure 94. Group mask project.

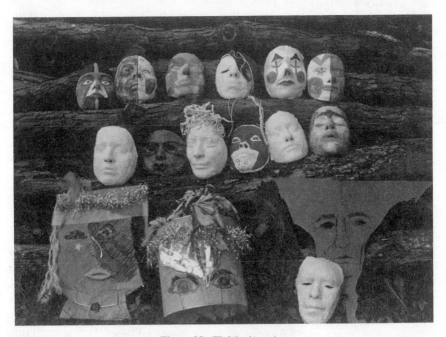

Figure 95. Finished masks.

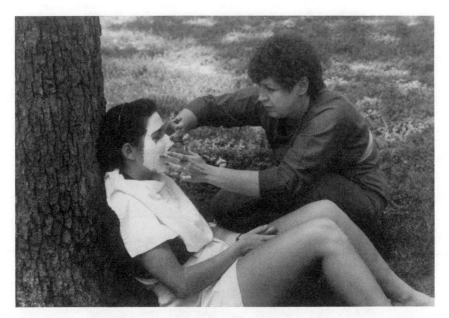

Figure 96. Gail Wetherell-Sack (right) pairs with Andy Kelinson in group mask-making.

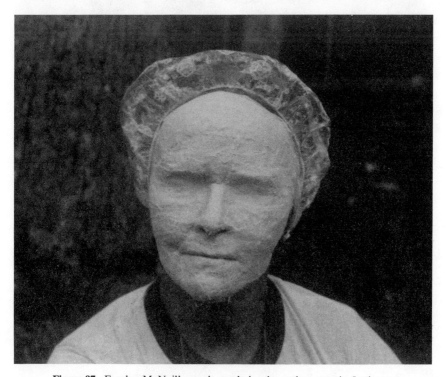

Figure 97. Evadne McNeil's mask, made by the author, sets in 5 minutes.

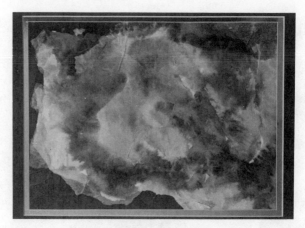

Figure 98. Tissue paper collage.

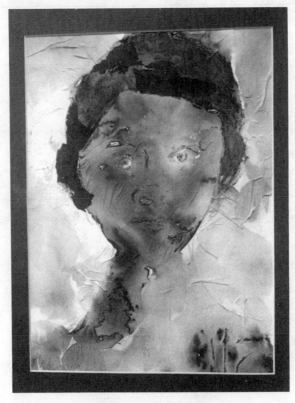

Figure 99. Tissue paper collage.

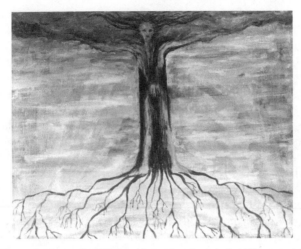

Figure 100. The author's acrylic painting of a woman/tree derived from a group art experience.

lead into the next, and observed their own progressions. Figures 98 and 99 were made by two of its members.

Figure 100 is an acrylic painting I created after a session in a group in which I painted two watercolors, one of a tree with an elaborate root system and another of a woman's face. They combined in this painting subsequently. In this sort of work, the group generally serves the purposes of stimulation, sounding board, and support for personal self-exploration and integration.

Art therapists who devote their working hours to helping their clients through art often neglect themselves. To paraphrase, we might say "art therapist, heal thyself." The communal sharing of image-making is one way to do so. Art therapists, in particular, find such groups especially rewarding, both as facilitators and as members.

NONINSIGHT ORIENTED GROUPS

There are groups for which neither the group dynamic approach nor the communal sharing of image-making apply. These are groups whose functional level does not allow for the development of much insight. Nevertheless, although some individuals do not function at a very high level, they may still be able to share a group experience, such as the "art club" formed at the Institute for the Study of Developmental Disabilities at the University of Illinois/Chicago. During her practicum placement there, Ellen Sontag established an art therapy program as part of ISDD's studies of the emotional difficulties of the mentally handicapped. The "art club" participants put on an annual art exhibit of drawings and paintings they made in art therapy at ISDD at the University. The members were obviously very proud of their works and talked about them at great length, despite the difficulty some of them had in communicating. The exhibit is now an annual event organized by each student in the placement. It is clear that not only is the art-making important to these people, but the sharing of it as well.

On the other hand, there are some patients who are so disturbed and self-absorbed that being in a group or participating with others is of little help to them. Nevertheless, art therapists sometimes find themselves in situations where they are obliged to see such patients in a group. Under such circumstances an open studio is a possible option.

OPEN STUDIO

The open studio provides an unstructured time when patients can make art at will. They may come and go as they please. The art therapist is there to facilitate what they want to do and they interact with her more or less as they choose. There may be little group interaction as there is likely to be no consistency in attendance. An art therapist may find it useful to provide open studio time in addition to regularly scheduled sessions.

SPECIALIZED GROUPS

There are many possibilities for specialized groups in addition to those mentioned previously. They may be more or less insight-oriented, depending on population, goals, and circumstances. Space does not allow for examples of all the different specialized groups art therapists might form. The following are two examples in which art therapists found creative solutions to difficult problems.

Gilda Moreno worked at a community center with a Hispanic population of chronic patients, some of whom had never learned to speak English despite living in this country for years. Gilda recognized that many of the patients suffered acculturation problems that were an intricate part of their emotional disturbance and poor functioning. To address this much

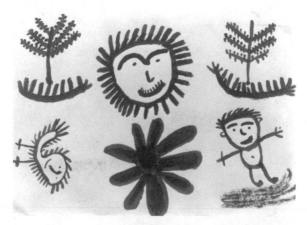

Figure 101. A picture from Gilda Moreno's group of Hispanic women.

neglected aspect of their dynamics she designed both an art therapy assessment procedure to identify the problems and an art therapy group to deal with the difficulties these people face. Most of the group members had lived in Chicago 10–15 years, yet their pictures related minimally to their current life situation. Figure 101, in vivid reds, was made by a withdrawn woman who spoke little and could neither read nor write. Her drawing depicts palm trees, a flower, the sun, a chicken, and herself. When she first came to the group, her drawings were pale and small. As the group developed, so did her ability to express herself through her art. The group's sharing of images of their countries of origin evoked poignant feelings and countered the isolation experienced by these chronically ill individuals who still felt like strangers in a strange land.

Figure 102 was photographed at a workshop led by Cherie Natenburg

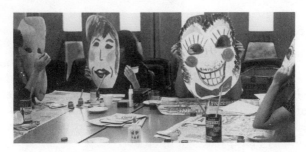

Figure 102. Communicating with masks.

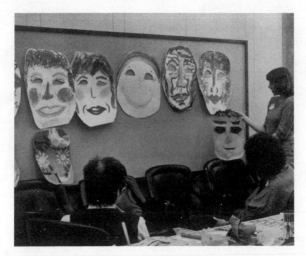

Figure 103. Display of masks with Terry Reimer discussing her mask.

in which she demonstrated a project she developed for the elderly with whom she was working. She cut out large paper masks for them to paint, offering an easy structured means for self-expression. In pairs they spoke to one another through their masks, telling each other what they saw in each other's face (mask). The masks were then displayed, Figure 103, so that all could be seen together and each could discuss his or her own mask. This exercise brought people more in touch both with themselves and with one another. As many elderly people are withdrawn and isolated, this exercise facilitated contact. The paired dialogue enabled people to speak to one other person's mask from behind a mask, thus easing the contact that may have been more difficult face to face.

CONCLUSION

In considering the many possibilities for group goals, composition, and structure, art therapists need to create a design that serves the purpose the group is established to meet. This is but one more enterprise that draws upon the art therapist's creativity. It is an area also where her confidence in her creativity may be challenged as others may try to impose a group art therapy design upon her.

Despite its complexities (or maybe because of them), group art therapy is often among an art therapist's most challenging and rewarding experiences. It is an area about which little has been written or demonstrated. Surely it is an area of work that looks forward to much creative development in new applications and ways of working.

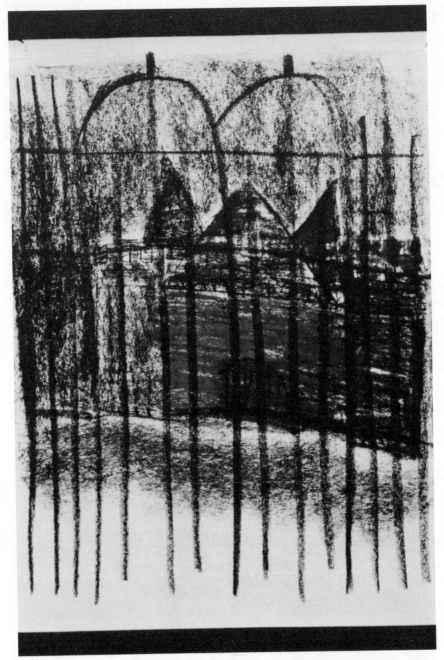

Figure 104. A delusion of the devil's castle by a schizophrenic young man.

PART THREE

Phases of Art Therapy

The art therapy process has a rhythm and a flow. It is important that art therapists be aware of the varied kinds of work required in the beginning, the middle, and the ending of a course of art therapy. Some art therapy procedures never advance beyond a beginning when art therapy is used for assessment purposes only. In ongoing work the beginning sets the stage for all that will follow. During the mid-phase much solid work may be accomplished. The ending provides the crucial work of dealing with separation, loss, and transition.

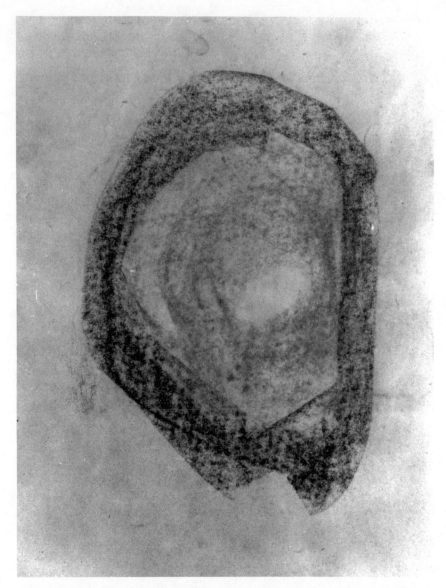

Figure 105. Entrapment in a picture of his marital relationship by a hospitalized depressed man.

CHAPTER 7

Assessment and Beginning Treatment

In a sense, treatment begins before the client or patient and art therapist even meet. The influence of what the art therapist brings to the encounter from her own development (Chapter 1), the nature of the therapy room and the art materials, and the method and source of referral (Chapter 2), all set the stage. Even more consequential is the larger context in which the art therapy is set (Chapters 10 and 11). The mission of the treatment facility and its methods plus the part art therapy plays in that mission are significant determining factors that shape the art therapy encounter before it has even begun. For example, art therapy in a school for behaviorally disordered adolescents that relies on a behavior modification approach is likely to proceed quite differently from a private group practice treating those same adolescents in a psychoanalytic framework.

Grounded in the context of her work, the art therapist may have some general goals in mind before she meets her client. In a crisis unit, she may want to help the client to take some immediate steps to handle the crisis. In a drug abuse program she may wish to ascertain if the client is aware of the extent of his problem. If there has been a significant recent loss, she may expect to help the client deal with anger and grief work. Sometimes a referral source will request a specific focus, such as dealing with body image.

In an institutional setting, the art therapist may read the patient's chart or the client's record for background information. I prefer to see the client initially free of bias in order not to be influenced by others' assessments in making my own. (We often tend to find what we expect to see and become distracted from other significant information.)

Assessment is part of treatment planning. Sometimes, however, an art therapist may conduct one or more sessions for assessment purposes only. Such is often the case in art therapy research protocols or to provide information for another therapist. For example, a psychiatrist in private practice requested me to see a chaotic family with whom he was working. He was interested in discovering if doing a nonverbal activity together might bring some order to their interactions (it didn't). Occasionally art therapists are asked to help verbal therapists who are "stuck." An example is the one session I conducted with a man hospitalized for psychotic depression and his wife. The psychiatrist and social worker who were treating them in couple therapy could get nowhere. The husband would not talk. In art therapy, however, he did communicate. His abstract picture of the marital relationship, Figure 105, in particular, facilitated the therapists' work with the couple. The husband was willing to speak about his picture, and said that in his marriage he felt trapped, enclosed, and surrounded.

Having digressed a bit, let's return to the consideration of whether the art therapist is conducting an assessment session or beginning treatment. She would approach each somewhat differently.

ASSESSMENT

The art therapist should be clear in stating to the client the purpose of the session. If it is to gather research data, she should not make a pretense of offering treatment. Nevertheless, it is certainly helpful to present the background information to the client in such a way that he will find the session useful as well. For example, when I was studying "The Marital Relationship in Manic-Depressive Illness," (Wadeson & Fitzgerald, 1971), I indicated to couples that they too might find the art exercises a new way of viewing their relationship.

Art therapists usually exhibit photographs of the art productions in research presentations and publications, thus it is advisable to give assurance about protecting confidentiality and to obtain release forms from the subjects. Also, the art therapist is better able to understand the context of the session if she knows what the payoffs are for the subjects for participating in the research. At the NIH where I conducted art therapy research for many years, patients received free hospitalization and treatment. Being there meant participating in whatever research was requested, including art evaluation sessions. Some were pleased to help in advancing scientific knowledge. Most responded positively to the interest I took in them. Art therapy there was certainly less invasive and frightening than some of the physiological procedures patients underwent. Some of the projects required that immediate family members participate in interviews as well.

In general, the art therapist's goal in an assessment session is to gain the information she wishes. A subsidiary goal is to establish rapport with the client. Unlike some other assessment procedures that can be forced (such as blood-drawing), art therapy requires cooperation. This is usually gained with a friendly, interested manner, empathy for prevailing concerns, and giving appropriate information and expectations. As part of the latter, some reassurance that there is no expectation of artistic excellence is helpful. I usually tell people that it's self-expression that we're interested in rather than artistic accomplishment and that I will rely primarily on them to let me know what their art expressions mean.

Generally, I try not to spend too much time talking. I give information, answer questions, establish some contact, briefly introduce subjects to the art materials and encourage them to begin.

If the assessment session is arranged in order to determine if the client is likely to benefit from continuing in ongoing art therapy treatment, then it is advisable to leave time at the end to discuss this, getting the client's reaction to the session and perhaps allowing him to be a part of the decision-making. Motivation goes a long way in effecting successful treatment. The first art therapy I ever undertook was set up on an assessment basis to determine interest in further treatment with the patients making the assessment. I established two groups of adolescents on a psychiatric ward. They were required to attend the first three sessions, after which they were to decide if they wanted to stay in the group or not. Even without art therapy experience, I recognized that adolescents who were forced into participating would rebel. But since they tended to be passive and negativistic, an initial push was needed. They all chose to remain in the groups (Sinrod, 1964).

Designing Assessment Procedures

Having introduced the gathering of information through an art therapy assessment in connection with structuring art therapy in Chapter 2, let's turn to a discussion of assessment development. The way to begin to design an assessment session is to think about what you want to learn and then develop the means for getting the information you need. Sometimes the latter entails reviewing the circumstances that have produced such information in the past. Often the best methods are the simplest and most obvious. When I was studying suicide, I asked patients who were hospitalized for attempting suicide to draw a picture of how they felt at the time. I learned much this way about their feelings of hopelessness, self-hate, entrapment (Wadeson, 1971, 1975).

When I joined a project studying acute schizophrenia, I was urged to design some research. I didn't know what to look for. I decided to get a feel for this population before plunging into questions that could turn out to be irrelevant. I would recommend this sort of decision to others. Research entails much too much work to spend countless hours chasing phantoms down blind alleys. For several months I met with the schizophrenic patients in art therapy sessions until I realized that what interested me most was their inner experience, not their behavior, reaction to medication, or whatever, but what it was like for *them*. In other words, my interest was in phenomenologically based research. It seemed to me that the most significant constituents of their experience of schizophrenia would be self-image, view of their illness, and hallucinations and delusions they experienced (the latter often being the determining factors in a diagnosis of schizophrenia). Figure 104 is an example of the latter. From an assessment that requested pictures of these phenomena, I wrote 14 papers.

Baseline Picture

As part of any assessment I conduct, I always begin with a "free" picture, that is, no instructions, whatever the client or patient wants to do. This way it is possible to observe the art expression untainted by expectations the art therapist puts forth. Once you have requested the patient to make a certain kind of picture or draw a certain subject, he is likely to believe that that is the sort of thing you are going to want from him. This expectation, then, is likely to influence other art productions. Sometimes it is interesting to compare what the patient comes up with on his own with what is a response to a request. One might be more fully developed or more controlled, for example.

In general it is best to keep exercises open-ended, leaving as much to come from the patient as possible. A request to draw one's family of origin is preferable to asking for a picture of one's father, mother, and brother. If I were the subject, I might also include the cousin who lived with us for most of my childhood and my cat.

Sometimes more information than meets the eye may be necessary in understanding an assessment. When asked to draw his family, a retarded child drew the family dog and no people, Figure 107. The school psychologist was concerned and showed the picture to the child's mother. She explained that the child's brother had just been given a dog whom he didn't want to share with his siblings. The parents repeatedly emphasized that this was to be a "family dog" for everyone to play with. The retarded child concretely attached the word "family" to "dog." The psychologist then asked him to draw the people he loved. He included all the members of his family, his teacher, and—yes—the dog.

Most of the assessment data discussed heretofore has relied on con-

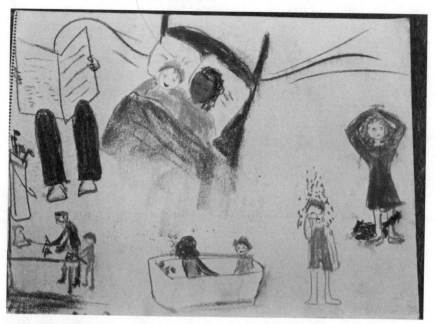

Figure 106. This family of origin picture shows scenes from childhood in which the patient (right) is isolated.

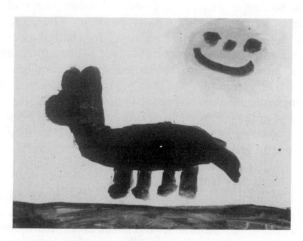

Figure 107. His "family" drawn by a retarded boy.

175

tent. Often other indices are considered. Ingredients of style may be telling in studying the effects of medication, for example. In attempting to determine "Characteristics of Art Expression in Depression" (Wadeson, 1971), I compared graphic attributes, such as color and utilization of space, during severe depression and when depression had lessened.

When research data is being collected, specific information is being sought. Assessment for treatment planning is another matter. Some art therapists like to use established procedures. When doing so, it is helpful to remember that there has been no standardization or empirical study of what conclusions, if any, such procedures yield. My assessment design is likely to consist of a "free" picture, something related to the reason for the client being in treatment (i.e., suicide attempt, drug abuse, the patient's reasons for seeking therapy), and whatever more flows. The assessment combines information revealed in the art woven together with its creator's responses to the art products and the art therapist's observations of the patient's thought, feeling, and behavior processes, in the context of any background or historical data that is available.

Assessment Pressures

It is important to recognize the context in which assessment often occurs, a context that reaches beyond the art therapist's research interests and treatment planning. Current trends in mental health and educational services require increasingly detailed documentation of treatment or educational objectives, plans, implementation, and results. Greater specificity is being required than in the past. Documented justification is often necessary for receipt of essential third-party payment. Thus, there is both greater dependency on and greater necessity for charted assessments.

Under these circumstances the art therapist is often pressured to produce a definitive initial assessment. How does she accomplish this? Often she grasps for a structure that will give her specific information, such as an assessment procedure developed and published by another art therapist. Since most of these assessment procedures have not been subjected to empirical evaluation, diagnostic conclusions drawn by their designers are not necessarily generalizable. Having developed several assessment procedures myself I am well aware of their limitations and the specific purposes for which they can be used.

A word of concern is in order here. For what future purposes the patient's record will be used, the art therapist often does not know at the time she adds her assessment to it. Decisions about institutionalization, discharge, medication, legal responsibility, and so forth, may rest on hospital, clinic, and school records. Even when the art therapist does not chart her conclusions, if they are presented at a staff meeting, they may be transposed to the patient's chart.

The point is not that the art therapist should refrain from assessing a patient, but rather that she should do so carefully and be willing to recognize that there is much she does not know or understand and that it takes time (beyond the initial interview) to gain a relatively full picture of the client and his problems, strengths, and situation. One must be open to additional information and the revision it may necessitate in the initial impression.

Despite pressures to the contrary, the responsible art therapist will chart in her assessment that some information was not obtained rather than coming to premature conclusions. Such situations are often extremely difficult, especially for beginning professionals. The desire for certainty is often strong and the discomfort with uncertainty, anxiety-provoking. Other staff members who often seem so sure of their assessments, may produce concrete data from psychological tests, and may expect the art therapist likewise to provide clearly defined assessment results. Although art therapists work in a field of especially rich data, its complexity often leads to its lack of specificity. One of the art therapist's tasks is to educate other staff members as to what might be expected from art therapy assessment and what is an unrealistic expectation. When specific information is sought, specific tasks to elicit that data may be designed, such as the suicidal feelings, hallucinations, and delusions, previously mentioned. In family assessments, people are often requested to draw pictures of their families (Figure 107), abstract pictures of family and couple relationships (Figure 105), and sometimes group or joint pictures in order to show interaction. On the other hand, if less-focussed information is sought, such as potentiality for committing child abuse, such information might not be evident.

In general, art therapists need to recognize and educate others to recognize that an art therapy assessment may produce an abundance of information, some specifically sought and some unexpected. On the other hand, the nature of the art expression may be such that it is impossible to draw substantial conclusions.

In sum, assessments are designed and conducted with the clear intention to gather information for one or more of the following purposes: clinical assessment for treatment planning or referral, determination of suitability of art therapy treatment, evaluation to obtain specific information, research. (For discussion of types of art therapy research, see Wadeson, 1980, Part VI.)

TREATMENT

As discussed in Chapter 5, one of the art therapist's most significant skills is in relating to the client sensitively and encouragingly so that much will flow, even in a first session. To begin that flow in ongoing treatment (even short-term), the art therapist's priorities are the reverse of those in an assessment. It is much more important to establish rapport than to gain information. She does so by being warm and friendly (though not effusive), interested, empathic, sensitive. She introduces the client or patient to art therapy in a way that will be comprehensible to him and hopefully not threatening. She is responsive to his feeling state. In extreme instances, this may mean dealing with delusional ideation. There are no formulas. She must try to meet the patient on his own emotional and cognitive ground. If he believes she's going to kill him, her suggestion of making a picture about it would hardly be an appropriate response. She may need to talk with him about it, show him that she has no weapons, and sit where he can watch her at all times. It is essential for the art therapist to grasp the framework from which the patient is operating. (Encouraging art expression and relating to the client are discussed in detail in Chapters 3 and 5.)

During the first session, the art therapist carries on a number of tasks simultaneously: (1) tries to establish rapport, (2) introduces art therapy, and (3) makes an initial assessment from which she begins to develop treatment goals and perhaps some methodology to implement them. Many of her interventions are in the service of more than one of these objectives. For example, at the same time that she is describing art therapy and giving the patient information about their meeting schedule, she is also establishing rapport and helping the patient to feel more at ease. Succinctly removing areas of uncertainty usually helps, such as, "We will meet every Tuesday from 10 to 11. I'll keep your art work in this folder with your name on it. From time to time I may meet with your doctor and show her your work or you can take any of it with you to your sessions with her whenever you want." To help people who seem uncomfortable to be more at ease with their discomfort, I often say something like, "Most people feel inexperienced in art and are uncomfortable when they begin art therapy." If sessions are tape-recorded or videotaped, I explain that too. I used to tape all my NIH sessions and explained quite honestly that no one ever has time to listen to them, including me, but that I taped anyway just in case there was something I would want to rehear.

Some people take notes. I have when I have needed direct quotes for research (I knew I wouldn't listen to the tape). But usually I find note-taking a distraction from giving the client my full attention. It tends to interfere with our rapport as well, erecting a barrier between us. I take time immediately following a session to jot down both concrete information and my reactions and assessments.

Having established the beginning of some rapport, given information about art therapy, and answered questions, the art therapist usually suggests that the client begin some artwork at this point. There may be exceptions, however. Sometimes I inquire about what brought the client to treatment and we talk together in what is usually a more comfortable mode of communication before I suggest artwork. In private practice, it is necessary to get some factual information as well, such as medication, insurance coverage, and so forth.

As previously mentioned, my first suggestion for art is a "free" picture, whatever the client wants to do. If there are "roadblocks," or resistances, they may have to be tackled, as described in Chapter 3. The art therapist's reaction to the first art expression is crucial. It sets the stage for subsequent processing. This most significant aspect of the work is described in Chapter 5.

Throughout all of the above, the art therapist is taking stock of her impressions, or "assessing." She may note that the client seems estranged from his feelings or that he is labile or that he appears to be hearing voices, or that he is trying very hard to please or that he is very sullen, and so forth. In addition to his behavior, his art may tell her that he is very disorganized, too preoccupied to invest more than minimal effort, or very meticulous, to name a few of the infinite possibilities. Further, the content of his art and his verbal elaborations may point up areas of difficulty such as loss, conflict, or low self-esteem, for example.

It is in the first session as well that the transference relationship begins to be formed. This is a particularly rich source of information. In this context, a therapist does well to examine her own feelings in response to the session. They will tell her much about the client. Was she bored, stimulated, titilated, angered, frustrated, confused, anxious, confident, relaxed? Ultimately, it is impossible to separate what you bring to the situation from what is the client's, but if you are sensitive to the different responses aroused in you by different clients, you may then get a handle on some of their interrelational dynamics. When the art therapist is aware of problems she is having with the client it may be helpful for her to examine what the client has aroused in her by processing her experience through her own art expression, as illustrated in Chapter 5.

A session has a flow and noting its direction also provides information. For example a patient may be extremely stiff at the beginning but soon relax, or pleasant initially and then become angry. The art may be defensive at first and then loosen up or start out disorganized and then become controlled; or the patient and his art may remain consistent throughout.

Some say that the central conflict appears in the very first picture. Throughout several years of art therapy a young woman wrestled with issues of longing to be my daughter and resenting my relationship with her "father" (psychiatrist). Her first drawing depicted a madonna-like woman holding an infant.

Figure 108 is another example of a first picture in which the salient issues for treatment are expressed. This picture was made by a young woman in a private practice group of well-functioning women. Toward the end of the group's life two years later, she reviewed her work and wrote the following about her initial picture:

> Lion Picture-Self Introduction: This is me in my favorite, gentle colors. I am aware that as I smile timidly, there lurks behind me, within me, a fierce, aggressive hating lion. I am afraid of him in me but want his energy and confidence. Above me flies a beautiful butterfly, delicate and full of life. I want to accept my beauty, inner and outer, and not be ashamed of it. These parts of me were not integrated when I drew the picture but now I am more whole. These parts were in conflict with each other and unacknowledged, although I was well aware of them.

The integration of the "beast" and dealing with the estrangement this dual experience of herself led her to feel proved to be her major therapeu-

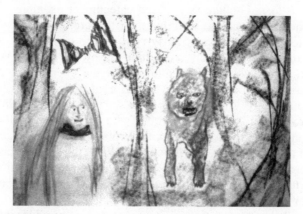

Figure 108. The first picture made by a young woman showing her split experience of herself.

tic effort. Her subsequent pictures eloquently made manifest the ego alien aspects of the "beast" and the separation from the rest of humanity she experienced in the "monster" that contained her, Figure 109. The art therapy process and the group support enabled her to integrate her experience, accept her previously disturbing feelings, and to feel more whole and less isolated from others.

It should not be assumed, however, that all first pictures are so revealing. People and their issues are much too complex to say it all in only one art expression. The art therapist must remain alert to the possibility of additional significant themes emerging during the course of treatment.

With all the aforementioned information in mind, the art therapist begins to plan treatment. This is an ongoing flexible process with new information added continuously and treatment modified accordingly. Planning includes both long-range and short-range goals, general objectives and specific strategies, all in the context of limitations and possibilities. The latter involve likely length of treatment, the client's ability to grow and change, support from the family if necessary (particularly important in working with children). Long-range goals might include such things as grief work or enhancing self-esteem. Short-range goals might focus on some immediate exercises for getting in touch with feelings. An example of a strategy, in contrast with the more general objective, was used in my work with a middle-aged man who had been in out-patient treatment for 24 years. He was the most anxious person I had ever seen. After the first couple sessions, I suggested he try some relaxation exercises. We continued to use them for the nine months we met, and he claimed they were the best part of the treatment.

In setting goals, the art therapist must be clear around what are her goals and what are the client's goals. Under the best of circumstances, they are identical. Some clients have no goals (except to get out of treatment) or their goals may be unrealistic (such as getting one's spouse to change). I try to be clear with clients about the differences and similarities in our goals. For example, an obese woman I saw in private practice asked me monitor her weight. I told her that my interest was not in helping her reduce but in working with her around her feelings of depression. I did not believe it would be helpful for me to be her task master. I also wanted her to be responsible for her own bodily functioning. The result was that as her depression decreased, so did her weight. Couples I saw in private practice often came with an agenda of "saving the marriage." I told them in the initial interview that such was not my goal but rather to help each to grow and to understand their relationship. Sometimes an initial session might reveal that the therapist's goals and the

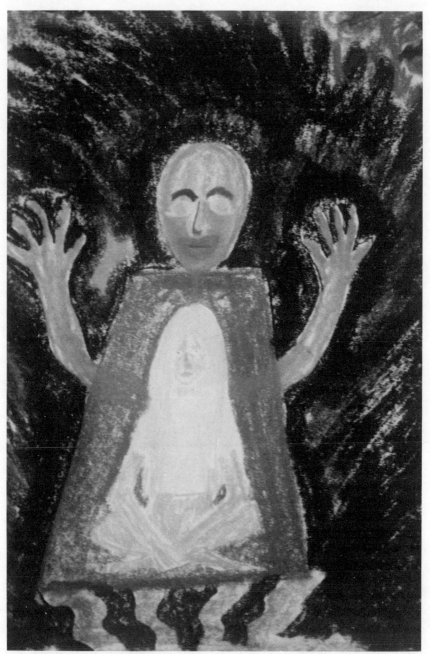

Figure 109. A self-depiction by the same woman who drew Figure 108.

client's are so different that they should not work together. Such was the case for a middle-aged couple who came at the wife's insistence in her effort to save the marriage. Her husband had already moved out physically and emotionally, and had agreed to therapy only as a result of her pressure and his guilt. Therapy was her last ditch effort to make him stay. I told her that I would not help her try to make him remain in the marriage. She chose to seek help elsewhere.

In most cases, however, the art therapy will continue. It is usually advisable to end the first session with some empathic or positive comment about the client's participation and a few words about the next session in order to offer encouragement and to establish continuity. I might say something like, "Even though you were reluctant at the beginning, I thing you really put a lot into your pictures. I'll see you next Tuesday." Since the first session often becomes something of a history-taking meeting at which many significant facts are collected, I usually make detailed notes right after the session, particularly about important points I think I might forget.

Beyond and including the first session, the beginning phase of treatment is a time for getting to know the client, for gathering information, for setting directions, for establishing a modus operandi together, and for the formation of the transference relationship. It is during this time that the significant issues for treatment will emerge. The art therapist begins to build a therapeutic alliance with the client, a way of working to be discussed more fully in the next chapter.

The beginning phase of treatment is crucial because it sets the stage for all the subsequent work. In short-term work, there may be little more than a beginning so that in some situations, it is the only phase of treatment as well.

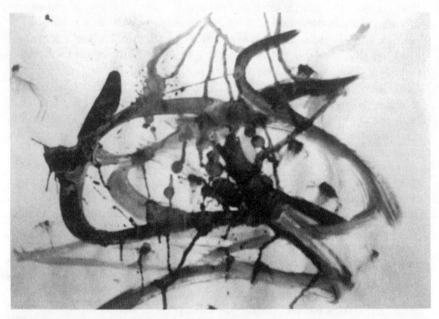

Figure 110. The paintings of a young man diagnosed paranoid schizophrenic were tight and controlled early in treatment, but several months later he was pleased with the freedom of expression he achieved here.

CHAPTER 8

Mid-Phase and Ending Art Therapy Treatment

MID-PHASE

It is difficult to determine when the beginning of treatment ends and the mid-phase begins. There is no clear juncture. In general, the honeymoon or initial "getting to know you" (which may be quite stormy and very "unhoneymoonish") has been completed and the art therapy pair has settled down to solid work. The "pair" refers to the art therapist and client, for that is what they have become. A large part of the initial therapeutic effort has moved in the direction of establishing a therapeutic alliance in which the two are joined in a task to deal with the client's problems. The dances around power, control, suspiciousness, and the struggles to test boundaries or limits have been resolved. Most significantly, trust has been established. The client knows that the art therapist is on his side in whatever wars he may be waging with himself or the world. At least, this is the ideal. Therapy is seldom smooth, so there may be set-backs along the way, but in general a method of working together has been established.

The manner in which all this has been accomplished is unique to each therapeutic alliance. In general, however, the art therapist is both firm and yielding. She establishes directions and boundaries—both personal and professional. She conveys consistent interest and care. She is receptive and accepting.

The development of the therapeutic alliance has required many meta-messages from the art therapist. She lets the client know that she respects him and is interested in him, that she takes his concerns seriously. She shows him that he can depend on her. If she says she'll be there Tuesday at 10, she doesn't show up at 10:15. If she says she will not allow him to throw paint at her and she can't control his doing so, then she calls an aide to help her. The client comes to know that she means what she says. He also comes to know that she says what she means. Her communication

185

with him is full and clear. I often share my strategies with my clients, and even more so once a therapeutic alliance has been developed. For example, I might tell a client that I will let him know when I am feeling distant from him, or angered, or whatever, so that we may examine what is going on. Or together we might develop a strategy. For example, I might say something like, "Since we've recognized that expressing anger is difficult for you, how about beginning with something small?" If he agrees, "What might be a situation where you have a small anger without large consequences for expressing it?" He might draw a picture of the situation to examine it and prepare for it.

The trust and confidence in the work that has been established allows greater freedom for the art therapist. Where there is sufficient ego strength, she can make interpretations without fear that they will be accepted because she's the expert or rejected out of hand as an act of rebellion. They can be used if facilitating or discarded if not. By this time the client has learned that it is not necessary to please the art therapist by agreeing with her. A beginning therapist, particularly, may have to deal with some of her own countertransference issues around the power a client gives her in trying to please her, in order to encourage the client's own self-determination.

The mid-phase is difficult to describe because it is at this time that the major issues are treated and the transference that has been established is utilized for treatment. Obviously, the issues and transference phenomena are unique for each client and patient.

The experimental aspects of art expression may have diminished as well, with the client settling into media he finds facilitating of his personal expression. On the other hand, there are some who continue to enjoy variety and may work in various media and styles. Additionally, the art therapist may suggest a different medium if the client appears stuck in an expressive rut.

It is rare during the mid-phase that I would use a preplanned exercise. My initial information-gathering structures are over (e.g., such as requesting a family of origin picture to obtain a history). The structure I would likely give the work might be occasionally suggesting that a client express in art what he is talking about (if he comes in recounting an experience, dream, fantasy) or perhaps for problem-solving purposes such as a picture of a job interview he is anticipating.

Examples

The following are a few examples of mid-therapy work: Figures 111 and 112 were drawn by a young woman suffering from colitus. After numerous physical tests, her physician referred her to outpatient psychotherapy for emotional causes, and I saw her in private practice. She was extremely conscientious at her job, frequently taking on more than her share of responsibility and working late into the night. Her illness so incapacitated her, however, that often she was unable to go to the office. She was offered a promotion but was afraid to take the position for fear that she would be too sick to handle the new responsibilities. Her treatment lasted approximately nine months and during the mid-phase she drew the two pictures illustrated here. Figure 111 is the pain in her gut looking like a red down-turned mouth. Figure 112 shows her stomach swollen and expresses her pain. During this portion of her therapy, she was able to identify her anger at her adoptive parents for continually threatening to return her to the orphanage during her childhood. She was also able to confront her own need to be "super perfect" at her job (so she wouldn't be abandoned by her "parents"). She recognized that she needed to work in a less self-demanding way. She also began developing friendships outside her place of work making it no longer the be all and end all of her existence. When she ended therapy, she was completely free of all the debilitating physical problems that had prompted it.

Figures 113 and 114 were made by another woman in the mid-phase of private practice treatment. In Figure 113 she shows herself in a "glass box" being scrutinized by her mother as she felt during her growing up, making her feel different from others. Figure 114 is a transference picture in which I'm drawn as an "exotic gypsy" with a "romantic castle" behind me. She is shown from the back, looking very plain in contrast. In fact, she was a very bright, beautiful young woman who saw herself as negatively "different." During the mid-phase she confronted many issues

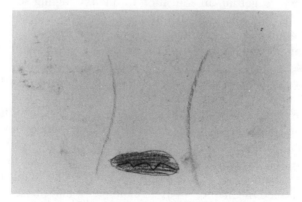

Figure 111. Pain in her gut by a colitis patient.

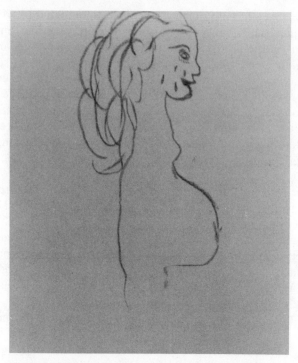

Figure 112. Sadness and swollen abdomen by the colitis patient who drew Figure 111.

around being a woman and feeling whole. Her treatment lasted several years, so during this time there were ups and downs, but she continued to make progress in getting an education through obtaining scholarships at the same time that she worked fulltime. Outwardly, she accomplished much, and gradually her self-image became more realistic.

In selecting examples of mid-phase pictures, it was not intentional that I chose self-images. Nevertheless, it is not surprising either. It is at this time in successful therapy that clients begin to recognize that their problems center around their views and feelings about themselves. The therapist can help them to question their perceptions and their attitudes. During this time, both these clients were able to see connections between parental treatment and present problems. They not only gained realizations in therapy, but began to apply them to make changes in their lives.

Figure 78, painted by Rachel—the 48-hour cyclic manic-depressive woman described in Chapter 5—is an example of mid-phase work with a

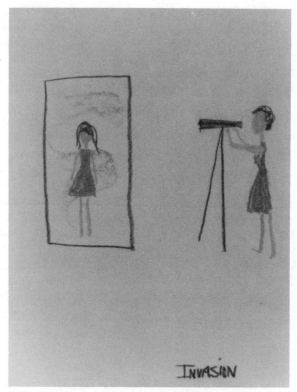

Figure 113. The client in a "glass box" being scrutinized by her mother.

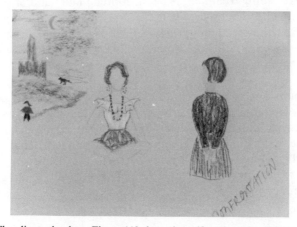

Figure 114. The client who drew Figure 113 shows herself on the right with the art therapist.

noninsight oriented patient. In her case, imagistic self-expression and a supportive empathic relationship were her gains from the art therapy. Initially, her manic pictures displayed grandiosity, anger, and high energy, while pictures made on depressed days were attempts at pleasantness. During both manic and depressed days of her 48-hour cycle (she had no in-between moods), her denial prevailed. During the mid-phase of art therapy, however, she became more in touch with her feelings and sufficiently trusting to express them. Figure 78 shows her being showered by her own tears. Such a strong expression of feeling was difficult for her, however, and she fell asleep several times while standing at the easel painting it, in what appeared to be an unconscious effort to avoid the pain.

The mid-phase is a time when the therapist's vacation might interrupt the work. (It is not likely that treatment would be initiated with a vacation about to be taken.) Naturally, the client should be told well in advance in order to have time to prepare for the separation and deal with the feelings involved. These often include anger, denial of anger, envy, and fear. Separations pave the way for the inevitable termination phase that follows. Sometimes, in fact, vacations are a rehearsal for termination. I have had patients in private practice realize during my vacations that they could live without me and thereupon initiate the termination phase. The separation serves a useful purpose in bolstering their confidence.

TERMINATION

Unlike the amorphous transition from the beginning phase to the mid-phase of therapy, the termination or ending phase is initiated abruptly and clearly. It is ushered in with an announcement by either the therapist or the client that ending treatment is being contemplated and/or planned. In a larger sense, termination begins in the first moment of therapy with the realization that the treatment is finite, even if open-ended, and will not last forever. Like life, if it were interminable, perhaps there would be no movement, no motivation to grow—why bother when there is an eternity to do so?

Separation is one of life's central experiences. Seldom is it possible to move to a plateau of greater growth without leaving a previous one. Separation constitutes some of life's most difficult experience, leading as it does to the realization for each of us of our own death. That most of us do not handle separations well is reflected in the dearth of writing on termination in the psychiatric literature. (As a result, I have included several references.)

The following is one of the most poignant descriptions of separation I have read.

Separation is inextricably bound up with that which in life we value most: growth, achievement, anticipation, the joyful sense of purposeful ongoingness. Yet each choice, each accomplishment, is a commitment, and further limits the possibilities of what can be . . . There is no joy that is not shadowed by its transience. There is no contact with another human being, no alleviation of loneliness, without the aching certainty—no matter how we try to hold it back—that loneliness will come again. No matter how desirable what is to come, it is yet unknown; and what is is sweet and terrible to lose.

In the pain of separation, man is confronted by the impermanence of his condition. Being and feeling are transient, in an indifferent universe, in which pain and loss are inevitable, in which change occurs without regard to one's own will or desire.

In our time we are faced not only by the inexorable catastrophes of nature that disrupt our lives with one pitiless disaster after another, by the meaningless accidents that mock us, and by the biological inevitability that dooms us to live in the shadow of continuous endings and final ending. But society, the structure by which man seeks to hold back change, to retain what is dear, to contain violence, and to give a semblance of order, permanence, and meaning—no matter how illusory—to the life he leads, is itself rent by cruelty, destructiveness, and upheaval. Human relationships, more and more, in a time of social chaos and dizzy acceleration, have a now, but a past that is brief, and a future that is uncertain and more often unlikely.

(Edelson, 1963, pp. 20–21)

TERMINATING TREATMENT

Successful therapy can reverse itself in the struggles to terminate, and what might have become a positive outcome may eventuate into a therapeutic miscarriage if termination is handled poorly:

The manner in which the therapeutic relationship is brought to a close is crucial to the outcome of treatment; it has a major influence on the degree to which the gains that occurred are maintained . . . Failure to adequately explore and work out these feelings during the ending period may result in a weakening or undoing of the completed therapeutic work

(Levinson, 1977).

To make matters even more problematic, it is characteristic that patients who have progressed well will begin to regress as the ending approaches, and many of the symptoms that characterized the patient's presenting picture will re-emerge (Levinson, 1977, p. 485; Dewald, 1971). The unknown is usually frightening, and the wish to remain in the present, known situation is often preferable to a future of uncertainty. Thus, patients are afraid to leave the support of the therapist. The more helpful the therapy, the more painful the leave-taking may be. Patients' regression toward termination time often conveys the message that they can't get along without the therapy. The understanding that termination regressions are expectable and not necessarily indications of major set-backs is an aspect of the process in which the therapist supports the client. Much discouragement can be avoided in this way.

There are a number of reasons for ending treatment, each one producing a different set of conditions and results. It is important that the therapist recognize these different conditions of termination, each of which imposes its various implications for the termination process. Termination may occur because the patient has completed therapy, is being transferred to another facility, or because the therapist is leaving the facility. Each of these situations differs from the other with regard to the feelings evoked. The termination of short-term therapy where there has been less engagement is likely to be considerably less consequential than termination from long-term therapy for both patient and therapist (Levinson, 1977, p. 481).

Termination from group therapy has further ramifications. The group, as a whole, may be ending and may have to deal with its dissolution. One member may be terminating, and the therapist will not only have to help that member come to closure, but also help the other members to deal with the loss of that participant (McGee, Schuman, Racusen, 1972). The group may continue after the therapist's departure, and she may need to help the group adjust to the transition as well as come to terms with her own feelings about not being indispensable to its life.

Because of the complexities and difficulties of termination the therapist should prepare the patient well in advance. This is done by bringing up the issue, focusing on its importance, and interpreting behaviors and feelings in the light of the pending ending (Dewald, 1971, p. 280). How far in advance this process begins depends upon the conditions of the treatment. In some instances, such as brief, time-limited therapy, it may be appropriate to point toward termination in the first session.

A further consideration in termination is the transference to an institution. It is both place and people. For patients it is often a home and a way of life. Termination requires leave-taking of that structure of support. Upon discharge, patients usually enter a world where they are expected to take on more responsibility, in a sense to become more adult. Although there may have been anger at the infantilization that patient status often encourages, there may be fear in having to become more responsible. Therefore, termination from therapy often necessitates attention to the institution's importance and what its loss means.

Just as elderly persons are encouraged to review their lives as it is approaching its end, so should the therapeutic endeavor be reviewed as it enters the home stretch. The therapist helps the patient to see what has been accomplished, what needs to be done, and points the way toward the future. If the nature of the therapeutic relationship has been mainly supportive, then the focus may be on how much the patient and therapist have meant to each other. There must be an acknowledgment of feelings of loss in any case, but also an emphasis that what has been gained has been a capacity to relate or engage, and that is not lost but can be utilized further.

Naturally in some cases there is bound to be disappointment and frustration at what has not been accomplished, which ending makes no longer possible in this particular treatment. These feelings usually must be acknowledged to produce a successful termination. If the termination process is painless, then probably little engagement has occurred.

Focus on ending often brings to mind other separations the patient has suffered. In this way, old angers and griefs are worked on and the patient is helped to deal with life's inevitable losses. It is this aspect of termination content and process that makes attention to its issues such powerful determiners of therapeutic outcome.

Because of its inherent painfulness, separation issues are often avoided, so there may be collusion between therapist and patient to avoid the processing. In this respect, denial often takes a strong hold.

Finally, it seems to me that just as a life process is seldom rounded out with a sense of completion—there is more left to be done—so it is with termination. There is always more to do in therapy. But there comes a time to end and to acknowledge ending.

TERMINATING ART THERAPY

With this brief overview of termination issues in mind, let's take a look at the unique contributions of art therapy to the process. To begin with, the client has created tangible products that he may take with him as reminders of the therapeutic journey or leave with the art therapist as pieces of himself in the hope that she will think of him.

The tangibility of the art products serves another terminating function as well. The art may be reviewed by the therapist, the client, or by both. I usually set aside time for the latter toward the end. This way the client and art therapist (and group members in group art therapy) can share a perspective of the entire art therapy process. Often times it is very gratifying and confirming to note the progress that has been made. Patterns that have emerged are highlighted as all the art is viewed together.

Finally, as expected, the art expressions provide an important vehicle for the expression of feelings around ending treatment and a means for saying goodbye. Often the art therapist participates as well, conveying through imagery her feelings about their separation to the client. These visual messages can be poignant and uplifting.

The encouragement to deal with attendant feelings about ending during this phase is often necessary. If the client is not doing so on his own, the art therapist may need to question his avoidance or to suggest that he examine such feelings in his art work. Figures 115 and 116 were drawn spontaneously by a woman hospitalized for depression and attempted suicide. "Bridge" connects the gap between hospital and home. She drew it in the context of "burning my bridges" as she prepared to leave but wanted this bridge to remain intact. (It turned out to be predictive as she was later readmitted following another suicide attempt precipitated by unusual stress).

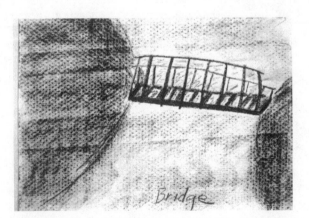

Figure 115. Bridging the gap between hospital and home.

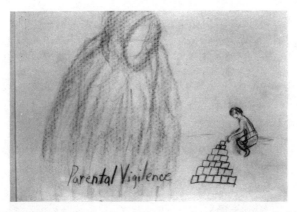

Figure 116. The hospital is watching over the patient as she builds.

In "Parental Vigilance" she depicted the hospital as a large ghost (perhaps related to her deceased mother) watching as she learns to build. This picture is particularly interesting as it resembles that aspect of the art therapy relationship akin to the attentive mother being present for her child as the child builds, creates, and learns. This is one of those ineffable characteristics of art therapy so difficult to describe. Small children often demand that their mothers watch as they draw or build or produce some other creation. Seldom in later life do we experience such devoted attention as we take on greater responsibilities in our lives. In art therapy, these early feelings may be rekindled as the art therapist is present for clients while they create. At termination of treatment the loss of that kind of love may be relived or experienced for the first time.

Hopefully, the client's terminating process deals with any grief, anger, disappointment, fear, hope, gratitude, affection, and confidence that may be present. One must bear in mind, however, that not all terminations from treatment are ideal. Some are aborted if the client leaves treatment prematurely or if a patient is transferred without warning. In other cases the denial is so strong that the feelings are suppressed. Usually, it is not only the client's feelings that are strong. The therapist must often contend with her own sadness, frustration, disappointment, or anger as well. Her own art processing can be especially helpful at this time.

In writing her master's degree thesis on the use of her own art-making to address countertransference issues, Barbara Fish described a particularly painful termination of a hospitalized patient with whom she was working. Barbara reacted strongly to the patient's decompensation and

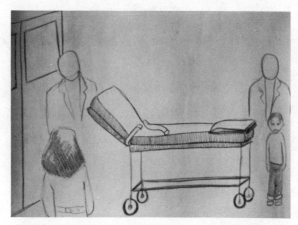

Figure 117. Art therapy student Barbara Fish examined her rescue fantasies and anger at other staff in her drawing of a patient's transfer to a state hospital.

her sudden transfer to a state hospital. Through drawing Figure 117, Barbara realized how some of her countertransference projections divided her from the rest of the staff. In this picture she has drawn herself in her hospital lab coat as part of the staff facing the ambulance cart and faceless attendants who are about to take the patient away. The patient, a middle-aged woman, is drawn as a child. Barbara wrote the following:

> My feelings of helplessness are illustrated through the powerful male figures, the locked doors and the ambulance cart. The cart elicits deep feelings in me about illness and powerlessness. These are feelings that I projected onto the patient. These may have intensified my discomfort with my inability to help her. When I look at this image I feel as though my child is being taken away. I think the patient's early developmental needs evoked a response from me that is similar to the symbiotic relationship of mother and child. This in turn evoked a countertransference response that relates to early nurturing experiences I have had. I am reminded of losing a doll. I felt punished, as if the staff had taken her away from me. My anger at the staff and the decision made by them is directed at the faceless male figures in this image. My feeling of helplessness opposed my clinical objectivity. I kept thinking that there was something I could have done to prevent her decompensation. I may also have been reacting to the radical psychiatric procedures performed on her in the past. She seemed so tormented, and I could not help.

Through her art-making and reflection on it, Barbara was able to address the anger and grief she experienced at the termination of this patient. In addition to ventilating her feelings, the art expression prompted examination of their emotional roots in this art therapist's early life experience and enabled her to work more effectively with other staff from whom she felt divided regarding this patient's discharge.

Art therapists are fortunate in that we have an expressive record of each patient's unique therapeutic journey in the artwork. I became more acutely aware of termination recently when I sold my house in which 15 years of patient art was stored. Looking through the pictures brought back memories of many people. Disposing of the artwork after all those years was a final termination. In that painful process, I realized how the art suspends separation a bit, how it enables people to leave a piece of themselves with another. When that too must be left, the art therapist who values those tangible expressions undergoes an additional termination.

The phases of art therapy are paradigmatic of much of life's experience. We touch another, we join, we create, we separate. Hopefully both partners, in this interchange take with them the growth they have derived from their shared experience.

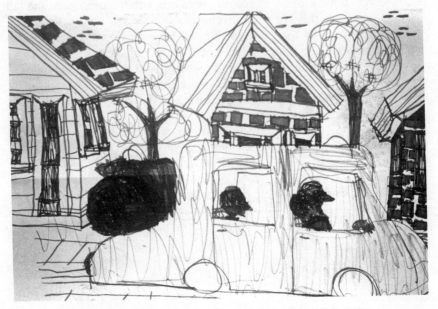

Figure 118. Dually diagnosed Dobie wanted to go home (I.Q. 34!).

CHAPTER 9

Examples of Phases in Art Therapy with Diverse Populations

In order to take a more comprehensive look at phases of art therapy treatment, work in some difficult settings will be presented to illustrate the nature of art therapy in various stages with diverse populations. As will become apparent, the problems, goals, and solutions vary considerably not only in treatment phases, but also among populations, settings, and even between individuals of the same population in a particular setting. Although there is no limit to the examples that might be cited, the following illustrations have been selected to provide a diverse range:

Developmentally delayed young adults treated for emotional difficulties in a university study program

A young woman jailed for the murder of her child

Chronic female patients of Hispanic origin with acculturation problems seen in a day treatment center

Formerly hospitalized patients with extensive psychiatric histories seen in a day treatment center utilizing a social rehabilitation model

An elderly physically impaired resident of a nursing home

Examples have been chosen to illustrate work with other than the usual in-patient and out-patient psychiatric populations that are discussed throughout this book and explicitly described in *Art Psychotherapy*. These examples have been selected as well to point up the wide range of application found in art therapy. Nevertheless, although length of treatment phase, problems, and specific goals may vary extensively, the basic considerations of each phase remain relatively constant.

THE DUALLY DIAGNOSED

In her master's degree art therapy training, Ellen Sontag was assigned a nine month internship at the Institute for the Study of Developmental

Disabilities Mental Health Program at the University of Illinois/Chicago. The Institute provides psychotherapy for persons who are mentally retarded and also experiencing emotional problems, thus the designation, "dually diagnosed."

Ellen found that much of the literature described this population as unamenable to insight-oriented therapy, yet her own experience contradicted this assumption. Because those with lowered intelligence levels are limited in abstract thinking and conceptual skills and often suffer language deficiency, they have been considered poor candidates for developing insight. For these same reasons, Ellen found that the concrete nature of art work can provide an avenue of self-processing and communication that may not be available to these individuals through verbal thinking and communication.

The intellectual, perceptual, social, and communication deficits of the dually diagnosed pose some unique problems for the art therapist. As the following examples illustrate, structural interventions during the various phases of treatment are often more directive in order to suit the client's level of functioning. End results are generally inferred from the client's behavior, rather than being directly communicated. Nevertheless, goals and results of treatment are remarkably similar to those in work with other populations (i.e., alleviation of depression, awareness, and communication of feelings, acceptance and mourning of loss, and improved interpersonal relationships). Levels of functioning, however, remain quite different from the general population. The following examples illustrate these results.

Tommy

Beginning Treatment

Tommy, a 14-year-old moderately retarded black male, was diagnosed as having antisocial behavior disorder. He had lived at a residential living facility for three years at the time of treatment. Tommy was referred to the ISDD clinic because of aggressive behavior toward people and property. He was also having trouble dealing with issues related to his family, as visits home were upsetting for him. Tommy's mother and stepfather disagreed over discipline, and his mother indicated that there was a lot of marital tension which seemed exacerbated by Tommy's visits home.

In his initial art therapy session, Tommy was immediately drawn to the paint and asked to use it. Ellen usually encourages clients to choose their materials, but the paint turned out to be overstimulating and disorganizing to Tommy. He worked without a baseline and began to paint objects and words in a chaotic manner. His behavior during the session became increasingly regressive. It was important to encourage a media choice that was less regressive in order for Tommy to use and build on to his already existing strengths. He entered therapy only too aware of his weaknesses and failures. This sort of intervention may be necessary in work with children or very disturbed adults. During the next session, Ellen offered markers, pastels, crayons, craypas, and colored pencils. Tommy chose to use pencil, probably the most controlled of all the choices. Within the framework of the more controlled media, Tommy began to draw a series of houses.

This became the theme that Tommy returned to at the beginning of each session for the next several weeks. Initially very shy and quiet, he began to share more verbally as he continued to draw houses. He had different family members living in each house, Figure 119. There was a lot of confusion about who lived in different houses and why. His biological father had left the family when Tommy was seven and had taken custody of Tommy's sister. Their loss and confusion over where his sister was, as well as why he had been placed in a group home, were themes that dominated these early sessions.

Tommy began to depict his perception of life's inconsistencies. At the same time (about six weeks into therapy), he began to question the tenuousness of his relationship with Ellen. Trust became an issue as he questioned: "Is this just our room?"; "Is anyone going to come into our

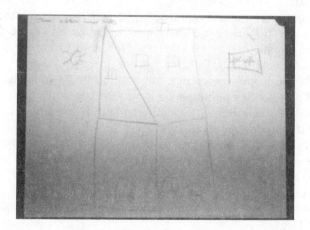

Figure 119. Dually diagnosed Tommy's house early in treatment.

room?"; "Would someone try to take our room away?" In response to his sense of vulnerability, Ellen made a sign with him that he insisted on hanging on the door. It read, "This is our art room. This time is for Tommy and Ellen and nobody can come in. Thank you."

Midphase

Tommy spent the next couple of months constructing houses from heavy cardboard and masking tape. His first attempts resulted in flimsy houses that couldn't stand up, but after weeks of working on the houses, they were larger and quite strong. For his last house, he constructed furniture and two people, his sister and himself. He was able to manipulate the people and furniture, and Ellen furnished a camera to take pictures of them. He was just beginning to untangle and mourn his loss.

Christmas vacation at home was a setback for Tommy and he returned more depressed. The next session was more like the beginning session, where he was not very verbal. He said in a very low voice, "I broke the bowl" (the gift he had made for his mother) and that he's "bad" because he breaks things and that's why he was sent to the group home. His mother related that he had also broken his brother's new toys and his own as well.

Clay proved a useful medium for dealing with his destructiveness. Tommy focused on the different ways that clay can be broken apart, and spent weeks breaking it. There were "rules" about this activity that helped to keep it safe for Tommy. For example, if he wanted to throw the clay, he had to confine it to the designated piece of newspaper for that purpose. After weeks of breaking the clay, Tommy began to use it to build. He made a Christmas tree which he reshaped into a lamp, Figure 120. As he did this, he talked about how, when he was home for Christmas, he was humiliated by his stepfather for being afraid of the dark. He had wanted the lamp on when he went to sleep, but his stepfather wouldn't allow it and teased him for wanting it. As he talked, Tommy again broke some clay and dumped it into the top of the lamp. Although Tommy initially had difficulty identifying and talking about his feelings, he was able now to talk about how angry he felt at his stepfather.

Tommy decided to paint the lamp and give it to the secretary at his group home. She was very special to Tommy and let him know that he is special to her. She hung the pictures that he made in her office. She placed the lamp carefully on her desk and appeared to reflect back to him the "good" side of himself. Subsequently he started to write "good Tommy" on his pictures.

Before giving away the lamp, he dumped out the broken pieces of clay

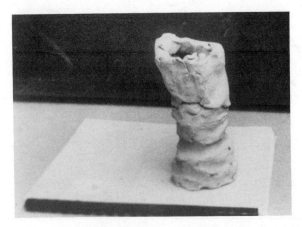

Figure 120. Tommy starts to build with clay.

that represent the part of him that is "bad," that breaks things. He wanted them wrapped up and placed in Ellen's desk drawer. It was important for him to witness their being locked up and for her to keep the key. The symbolic nature of this act was of considerable import to him.

After almost three months of working with clay, Tommy returned to drawings of houses. These houses were larger and better organized than his initial drawings (Figure 121). He began to verbalize more again, and enjoyed making up stories about the houses.

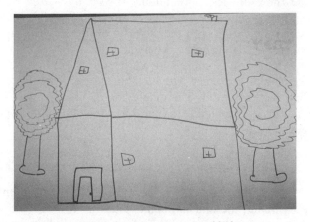

Figure 121. Tommy's house in mid-phase.

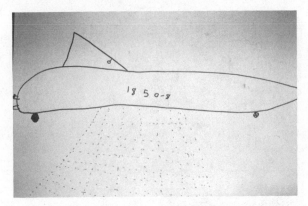

Figure 122. Tommy wants to drive away at termination.

Termination

Tommy's reaction to Ellen's announcement that she would be leaving ISDD was to become guarded. He announced that he was moving tomorrow and wouldn't be back next week. In this way he could do the leaving rather than be left as he had by his family. He spent several weeks talking about moving and drawing cars driving away (Figure 122).

Results of Art Therapy

Tommy was not very verbal and was initially very shy. The art therapy offered a means of developing a relationship that was less demanding verbally and therefore less threatening to Tommy. Often "out of control," manipulation of the materials gave him a means of developing more control. In experimenting with the clay, he examined both sides of himself. He saw the side that broke things and the side that created things.

The concreteness of Tommy's artwork was useful to his relationship with the group home secretary. He was able to offer something of himself, which she in turn treasured. The displaying of Tommy's artwork in her office was a constant reminder to him that she valued him. This enabled him to begin to value himself.

Dobie

Tactics in the various phases of art therapy were quite different with this client. She exhibited the unusual combination of low IQ (34) and almost complete lack of verbal ability with extraordinary skill in art-making.

Dobie was a 21-year-old severely retarded black female who had lived in large state institutions since she was eight. She demonstrated aggressive behavior toward herself and others and frequently masturbated with a chair or hairbrush. The masturbation was extremely self-injurious. Other problem behaviors included scratching and slapping others and the destruction of property.

Dobie's family had maintained a caring relationship, often taking her home for months at a time, until approximately two years previously. At that time the family underwent personal problems that resulted in their no longer being available to her.

Beginning Treatment

Dobie began initial sessions by saying "mama," her sister's name, or mentioning McDonald's. Through these initial sessions, Dobie drew scenes of herself at her mother's or sister's house. She portrayed herself doing the things that she always enjoyed with them, although she hadn't seen them in two years. She never drew a picture of or spoke of the staff or residents at her living facility or the workshop where she worked.

Dobie would ask for cookies at the beginning of each session and refreshments became a ritual for beginning sessions. This lasted throughout art therapy. During those early sessions, Dobie continued to connect mama and sister with the nurturing she needed. Session after session would start with the naming of mama or sister and some associations with foods that she liked such as McDonalds, Brown's Chicken, Cheerios, and french fries. These were some of the special treats that she received at the living facility. However, she was not yet ready or able to acknowledge that these needs were being met by others who cared for her.

Dobie presented an initial theme that dealt with her need for nurturance from her family, and her confusion and feelings surrounding the loss of her previous relationship with them. As Thanksgiving approached, Dobie began to act in a more anxious manner. She drew a picture of her sister coming to pick her up for Thanksgiving. She added a huge bundle of belongings to the car, indicating that she intended to stay for a long time (Figure 118).

Midphase

In order to give Dobie a way to express some feelings, Ellen attempted to teach her to identify and label "happy," "sad," and "mad." She drew pictures of different faces and labeled each with a feeling. She and Dobie practiced making the faces while looking in the mirror. Then they talked about different situations and how they would make them feel. Dobie identified herself as feeling mad if she didn't go home. Then she spontaneously drew her own face. This was the beginning of being able to identify and verbalize simple feelings. These pictures were used in many future sessions to help express feelings.

As Christmas vacation approached, Dobie again exhibited a lot of anxiety about going home for vacation. As she had not gone home for Thanksgiving, she was now worried about not going home for Christmas. She drew pictures with herself "phasing out," a comment on how she felt her position in the family was changing. In Figure 123, Dobie drew Mama, her sister, and another family member in a large, detailed way. She included herself in the picture much smaller, and so darkly colored that no detail is apparent. Compared to the three other figures, she barely exists.

Another manifestation of Dobie's anxiety was her increased acting-out behavior. Some of the behavior that had previously been problematic returned for the first time since she had started art therapy. She became aggressive toward staff members and was 45 minutes late one week because she had attacked the staff member who was driving her to the session. She again became quite destructive, smashing the fish bowl and throwing the TV in her living unit.

Ellen worked with the faces that she had made to help her identify and communicate feelings. Ellen suggested that maybe she was again worried that she would not go home for vacation. Dobie acknowledged this, choosing the angry face to further express her anger at the possibility of not returning home. She then drew a picture of herself throwing the TV

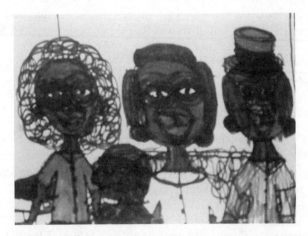

Figure 123. Dobie appears insignificant in her drawing of her family.

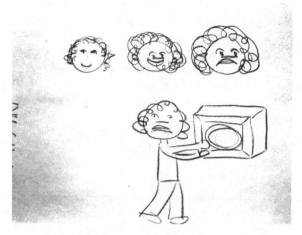

Figure 124. Dobie's anger.

and said, "Angry throw the TV" (Figure 124). She followed that by drawing the TV in the living room at her mother's house saying "Go home" (Figure 125).

In this way, Dobie was able to use the pictures and simple words to communicate her feelings. After that session, her acting-out behavior diminished. She was beginning to incorporate alternative ways of coping and expressing feelings.

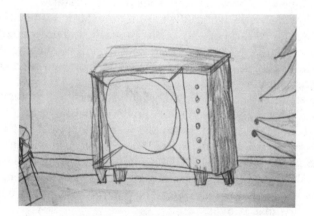

Figure 125. The TV in Dobie's mother's home.

After Christmas vacation, Dobie seemed resigned, but more accepting of the changed situation at home. She announced "Christmas is over," "Mama and sister are gone." For the first time Dobie began to speak about other people, for example a staff member who had fixed her hair and another who had given her a sweater for Christmas. She was beginning to integrate other people into her life.

For the next two months, Dobie chose to work with clay to recreate her mother's and sister's houses. She kept these clay pieces on her dresser where they served as icons. The art helped her to accept the loss of her family but retain them symbolically.

Termination

The termination work reinforced all the work that Dobie had done in art therapy and demonstrated her remarkable ability to communicate visually. For the last six weeks of treatment, she made a weekly picture around a single theme to enable her to integrate her therapist's leaving.

Ellen told Dobie that she was a student who was graduating, and that in June it would be time for her to leave ISDD. She helped get these ideas across by drawing pictures of the calendar months and naming them with her. June was discussed as being the beginning of summer in order to give Dobie some sense of time left. In response to Ellen saying how important the meetings had been to her, Dobie said, "Dobie mad." Ellen asked, "Do you mean sad?" She said, "No mad!" Dobie was now able to distinguish and express feelings, her insistence that she was "mad," not "sad." She then said, "Christmas is over." She was remembering the painful feelings of separation from someone important.

The following week, when Ellen again brought up termination, Dobie replied, "Summer, carnival, fun." She proceeded to draw a ferris wheel ride. The next week, she merely said "carnival" and seemed anxious to begin work. She made an enlarged picture of a merry-go-round and again said, "Christmas is over."

Ending each session with Dobie became increasingly difficult. Her behavior didn't have an oppositional, stubborn quality; as she was told it was time to stop, she continued on. She seemed to have a real need to get some information down on paper. When Dobie arrived the following week, she said, "Go carnival" and wanted to start drawing immediately (Figure 126). At each session, she drew a carnival scene. At one she said, "Go home for Christmas?" Later she answered her own question by saying, "Christmas is over."

At the next-to-last session, she placed herself in front of the merry-go-round. The self-portrait is sturdy and strong. It lacks the stereotyped face

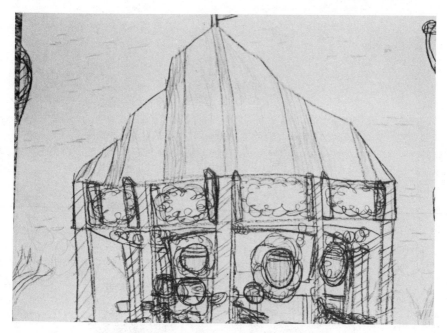

Figure 126. Dobie's carnival termination picture.

with a smile that she characteristically drew in earlier drawings. There was a peacefulness and strength both to the drawing and to the session (Figure 127).

Her last picture also includes herself. The figure on the left is Dobie, and the one on the right is Ellen. The two people are working together to run the ferris wheel (Figure 128), metaphorically describing their working together.

Results of Art Therapy

This almost nonverbal woman with an IQ of 34, who had been institutionalized for most of her life, made some impressive gains. She was able to develop a significant relationship with her art therapist and become aware of her own feelings and identify and communicate them. Most important, she came to terms with her present life situation, accepted the loss of her family and utilized this integration in effecting a positive termination of her treatment and separation from her art therapist. Certainly, for this handicapped woman, her remarkable ability in art was a strength worth tapping for the potential it provided her for self-awareness, integration, and communication.

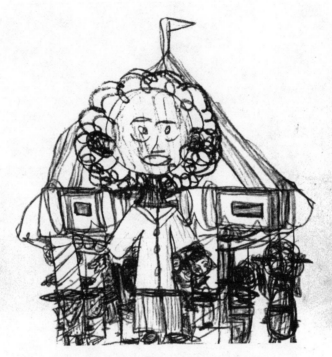

Figure 127. Dobie at the carnival.

Therapeutic Phases for the Dually Diagnosed

In work with the dually diagnosed, beginning art therapy must usually entail an assessment of the client's functional and art abilities. As in the case of Tommy, interventions are sometimes needed to preclude art activities that might not be beneficial (his choice of paint that was too chaotic for him at the time) and to suggest media that would facilitate growth. Engagement often necessitates concrete assurances, such as the sign Tommy hung on the door to secure his time and place with Ellen.

As in therapy with other populations, it is the mid-phase, after engagement has been established and trust built, that much of the major therapeutic effort is accomplished. Both Tommy and Dobie dealt with loss. Tommy discovered that he is "good" and can create, as well as destroy, which had made him feel "bad." Dobie learned to recognize and articulate her feelings.

Termination, often difficult and at times unsuccessful, poses special

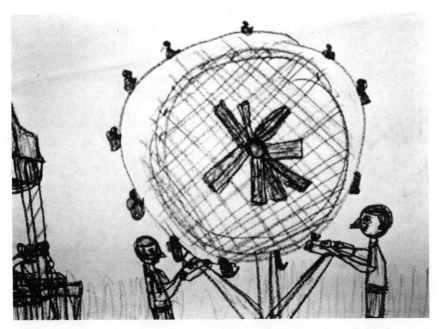

Figure 128. Dobie's final image of the carnival, operating the ferris-wheel with her art therapist.

problems for the dually diagnosed. Often they have suffered losses that they do not understand, resulting in confusion, anger, and depression. The ending of their art therapy sessions and the reasons for their therapist's departure are often incomprehensible to them. It takes great effort and skill on the part of the art therapist to effect a positive separation. Tommy withdrew and fantasized that he was leaving rather than being left. Through her art, Dobie appeared to accept Ellen's leaving and further integrate the loss of her family. Her final picture was an eloquent statement of how she and Ellen had worked together as equal partners.

INCARCERATION

To pursue her interest in criminology, Rose Marano Geiser interned at Chicago's Cermak Jail during her master's degree training at the University of Illinois/Chicago. She worked in the jail's psychiatric services on both men's and women's units. Psychiatric care was oriented primarily toward crisis intervention as inmates remained for indeterminate periods of time depending upon court disposition. For the most part, the jail is a holding facility prior to inmates' trials that may direct transfer to a prison or to a hospital psychiatric unit.

For nine months of her incarceration at the jail, a woman who had shot and killed her four-year-old daughter was seen in art therapy. The nature of her crime was a significant challenge to Rose in sorting through her own feelings about the murder of a child. She first saw Terry at her initial intake interview conducted by a mental health specialist. Terry remained silent and refused to answer questions. She was placed in the jail's acute psychiatric unit for observation and assigned to a pediatracide group for woman accused of child abuse and infantacide and to an art therapy group. In both, Terry remained silent and withdrawn. As a result of her passivity in these groups, she was referred for individual art therapy.

Terry was a 28-year-old white high school graduate from a working class background who had taken a few college courses and worked for two years as a cashier in a food store. This was Terry's first incarceration, and there was no history of previous hospitalizations or prior mental health treatment. She had been married, had one child, was separated from her husband because of his physical abuse, and moved with her child to live with her parents. Also living there were her older sister and her identical twin.

Beginning Individual Art Therapy Treatment

With an indeterminate treatment period for which to plan, Roses's goals were to help Terry understand her feelings and deal with her present difficult situation. Additionally, in order to be able to help her patient, it was necessary for Rose to come to some understanding herself of Terry's crime and to be able to come to a nonjudgmental acceptance of Terry.

At her first individual session, Terry was initially cheerful but then became tearful as she discussed her drawing of her daughter. She spoke of not wanting to have a child and being disappointed that the baby was a girl, yet described her daughter as central to her life. Apparently the four-year-old had regressed to the "baby stage" when Terry and her husband separated. Terry recalled being afraid she would hurt her child and locked herself in the bathroom whenever these hostile feelings arose. Terry was angry that her family did not take her seriously when she told them of these feelings. In this first session, Terry described some of her ideation leading up to killing her daughter. She was afraid that her older sister would take her daughter from her or that the child would be placed in a foster home where she would be beaten and raped. In order to prevent this from happening, while distracting her daughter with a toy, Terry shot her. When the gun fired, she could not believe what was happening because she had thought the gun was not real. As the child cried out, Terry knew she would have to kill her because now her child would surely be taken away and would never overcome the trauma of being shot by her mother!

Having told her story, Terry stopped crying and spoke of how relieved she was to have told someone what happened. She was afraid to talk to the inmates on the women's tier where she had been placed because of what she felt they might do to her for the crime.

This first session was obviously one of major catharsis and almost immediate trust building. The art therapist was presented with a great deal of data, much of it contradictory and confusing, reflective of the patient's confusion and ambivalence. As Rose helped the patient to untangle her feelings, it was necessary for her to do likewise in sorting through her own reactions.

A couple of sessions later, Terry drew a dream in which she was pregnant a second time and described herself in the dream as being hysterical in not wanting a new baby, but wanting her now dead daughter (Figure 129). She spoke of her feelings during pregnancy. She had planned an abortion but was talked out of it by her sisters. She reflected: "It was inevitable that I killed her, it was only later. It didn't matter." Intense feelings and lack of feeling followed rapidly upon one another.

Midphase

Throughout her treatment, Terry continued to express marked ambivalence toward her daughter, including much projective identification. At one point she related contemplating suicide but not wanting to endure the physical pain of shooting herself. She spoke of not having to feel the pain in shooting her daughter, but with the child's first cry realized the pain she was in and had to kill her to stop the pain. She now felt the child was at peace and that God had intended her to shoot her daughter, otherwise he would not have allowed her to do so. She was obviously trying to find ways to release herself from blame.

During this period she also dealt with her feelings about her life in the jail and was relieved that her psychiatric evaluations in the jail determined that she was schizophrenic. This would influence sentencing in favor of hospitalization rather than imprisonment.

Most significant in her work was her attempt to explore her family relationships. There was much competition with her twin sister who underwent several psychiatric hospitalizations and ran away during Terry's

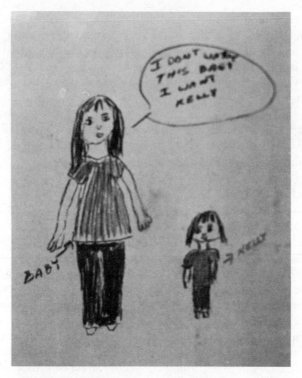

Figure 129. Jail inmate Terry's dream of being pregnant.

imprisonment. Terry was resentful that her parents seemed more concerned about her twin than about her at this time. There was also resentment toward her mother-in-law who was a dependent person whom Terry described as wanting to be taken care of by others. Terry resented her for being able to leave the house while Terry had to remain home and take care of her daughter.

Of particular importance was Terry's rivalry with her daughter for her place with her sisters. In Figure 130 Terry has drawn herself on the left at the kitchen table with her sisters. She reminisced about the rugby team they played on together and how they would sit together in the kitchen discussing the games. These talks stopped when she moved back into her parents' house. Her sisters then played with her daughter "all the time" and talked about Terry with their father and would stop "whenever I entered the kitchen."

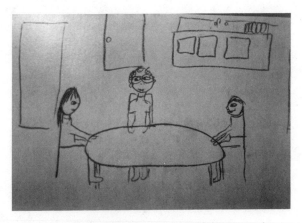

Figure 130. Terry and her sisters.

Termination

As is usually the case in work with jail inmates, the termination phase is related to trial dates, rather than either the therapist's leaving or completion of treatment. Rose had discussed the time when the sessions would end during the initial sessions of treatment, and as Terry's trial approached, termination issues surfaced readily. These issues centered appropriately on her anticipations and concerns about her uncertain future and her relationship with Rose and separation from her.

In Figure 131 she drew her expectations of transfer to a state mental facility, having been assured by her lawyer that he would win his plea of insanity. Her associations were fears that other patients would find out her crime, that she would be raped by male patients, and that she would be unable to resist her own sexual desires. In the middle level of the picture, she is lying on a doctor's examining table and sitting in a dentist's chair. She spoke angrily of hating to be probed.

As her court date drew nearer, Terry expressed her anxiety in a courtroom picture, Figure 132. She is seated on the right, crying. She spoke of dreading the trial because she would have to hear all about the crime again.

As Terry expressed anger at the jail, Rose suggested that perhaps Terry was angry at her. She assented readily explaining that she was angry that Rose could leave any time she wanted and that she could not help her get out of jail. She claimed that she needed more frequent sessions and in her ambivalence, spoke of feeling safer in jail than outside.

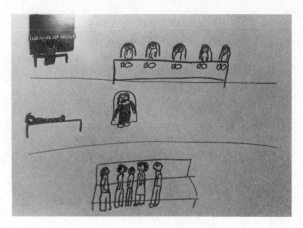

Figure 131. Terry's expectations of transfer from jail to a state mental facility.

Terry drew her relationship with Rose in Figure 133. Terry is on the left with the balloon above her head showing her daughter and sisters, "what we talked about most." Terry indicated that the balloon's blank area represents all the "bad things" she left out. She spoke of having told Rose more than anyone, "more than my sisters," but the blank space indicates how hard it was to trust anyone in revealing her feelings. She noticed that in the picture Rose's back is "awfully straight" and connected it with a lack of trust on Rose's part as well. She suspected that Rose did not like

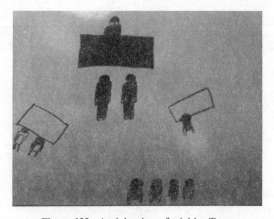

Figure 132. Anticipation of trial by Terry.

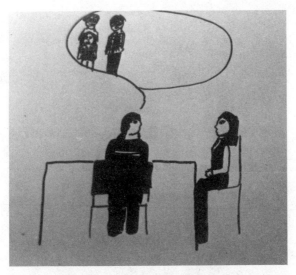

Figure 133. Terry's relationship with her art therapist.

her and that no one could for what she had done. Rose assured her that although she did not like her crime, she liked Terry as a person and had felt touched by their sessions together.

Figure 134 was Terry's final picture made during the week of her trial. She said it looked frightened and mad. She thought the eyes probably resembled the look she had after shooting her daughter. She and Rose discussed the loss of people she loved and that they would not work together in the future.

Two weeks remained for both Terry's and Rose's stay at the jail. Terry had learned that she would be transferred to a state mental hospital. During this period she refused further art therapy sessions on the pretext that she was too busy. It appeared that looking into her crime and herself further and separation from Rose were more than Terry could handle. More often at the jail, Rose was confronted with abrupt patient transfers, cutting off therapy before a termination phase could be completed.

Results of Treatment

The jail is a holding facility pending trial and transfer. Treatment therefore, is of much the same nature. Clearly Terry had only begun much-needed therapy. The beginning phase was a dramatic catharsis for this young woman who was suddenly overwhelmed and confused by her own

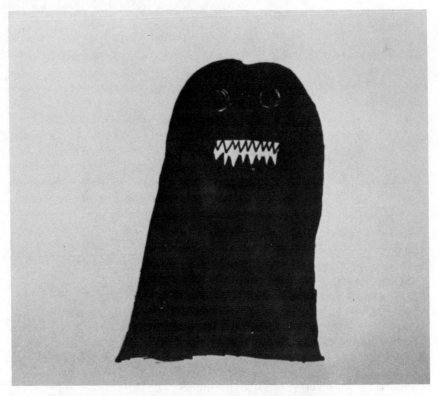

Figure 134. Terry's final picture associated with her murder of her child.

destructive act. In a jail setting that can be frightening and dehumanizing and with an impending trial that is often extremely anxiety-provoking, engagement is of great consequence.

During the mid-phase of work, Terry scratched the surface of problematic family relationships and dependency needs, indicating areas for work, but was not at a point where integration could begin. Clearly, she is a patient for whom long-term therapy is needed.

Termination centered primarily on trial and transfer anticipation as these were the enormously consequential real-life events with which jail prisoners must contend.

Art Therapy in a Penal Institution

Work in a penal institution poses significant challenges to an art therapist. Extreme security precautions are necessary; inmates often have a history of violence; trust may be difficult to develop; the system of incarceration itself may be dehumanizing; depression and anxiety are often pervasive, and suicide may be a prevailing threat. Not the least of the difficulties is the art therapist's task in relation to people who have committed acts she finds heinous. In Rose's case, her initial discomfort with Terry's murder of her child was supplanted by feelings of care and fondness for this confused young woman. Rose came to recognize that Terry's boundaries between herself and her child were blurred and that in the actual murder she did not seem to know what she was doing. The task of joining patients emotionally when their behavior is so ego alien to the therapist is nowhere more pronounced than in work with criminal populations.

ACCULTURATION PROBLEMS*

In work with an immigrant population, preparatory work is necessary in advance of therapy. At the most obvious level, language may be a problem unless the therapist is bilingual. Less obvious is the need for the therapist to be bicultural as well. As a Cuban refugee to this country, Gilda Moreno requested an internship at a facility serving Hispanic clients. In preparation, she reviewed the literature and integrated the findings of sociological research with her own migratory experience in understanding the problems of her clients.

Reports in the literature indicate that Hispanics, the second largest minority group in the United States, have been resistant to engagement in a therapeutic relationship. Lack of availability of culturally sensitive services in the Hispanic "barrio" (neighborhood) is often part of the problem. More significantly, however, Hispanic family structure often mitigates against seeking help outside the family.

The population with whom Gilda worked at a Hispanic neighborhood community mental health center was composed primarily of female chronic patients who had immigrated during adolescence or adulthood and had lived in this country for five or more years. Some had been coming to the clinic for 10 years. Most were poorly educated and spoke little or no English. Typical of Hispanic family patterns is a rigidity of sex roles in which the wife devotes herself to her family with the husband and children having greater contact with the community. As a result, the women are often isolated from the host culture in addition to being cut-off from country and family of origin.

---

* This material is presented in greater detail in Moreno and Wadeson (1986).

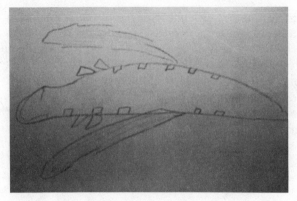

Figure 135. An Hispanic chronic patient wants to return to Puerto Rico.

Assessment

In order to assess the interplay of acculturation problems with the women's psychiatric condition, Gilda developed an assessment procedure consisting of four drawings: a free picture, a memory from life in your country of origin, something significant from your life in Chicago, something or someone from your country of origin you would like to have in the United States. The results brought forth memories from childhood and showed little attachment to life in Chicago. For example, Figure 135 is "something significant from your life in Chicago," a plane leaving O'Hare Airport for Puerto Rico. Complimenting the lack of investment in life in Chicago, the fourth picture revealed a longing for both people and place from the countries of origin.

The art therapy assessment was used as a part of the intake procedure and in many instances aided in diagnosis and identification of significant issues for treatment planning and therapist assignment.

Beginning Treatment

An ongoing art therapy group was formed with new members added as they entered the treatment center. The group met for 20 sessions over five months with membership fluctuating from four to six. Because the population was a chronic one, the atmosphere was designed to be relaxed with no tasks assigned nor pressure applied to urge members to discuss their art. All sessions were conducted in Spanish.

Collage-making was an especially comfortable activity in the group's early stages because it involved a series of steps compatible with the

Hispanic way of socializing. The group would peruse magazines together and share pictures with one another. This led to an increased discussion of the themes that emerged. Figure 136 is a collage made by Ileana, a 27-year-old woman who had lived in the United States for eight years. She was referred to the clinic because she had been physically abusive toward her child, who was eventually removed from the home and placed with the maternal grandmother for protective custody. The collage shows the clothes of which Ileana is very conscious, her "dreams" for a beautifully decorated home, and toys for her little girl.

Midphase

Reunification with her child and her extended family remained Ileana's goal throughout therapy. In Figure 137, she depicted herself with her family in Puerto Rico. Through her art, she was able to visualize and later verbalize her hopes and what steps she would need to take in order to attain them.

A frequent group topic was the difficulty of adjustment to the cold. Drawings often depicted life in a warm climate with images of palm trees, fruit, the sun, and the sort of houses found in the Caribbean islands.

The group became a safe place where its members could share with one another the hardships of their present life situations and reminisce about their lives in their countries of origin. As they drew and discussed their conflicts, they interrelated and became very supportive of one another. This was an important step for those relatively isolated individuals. The recognition of the universality of their shared migratory experience was of significant support. For women who had been acculturated to put their

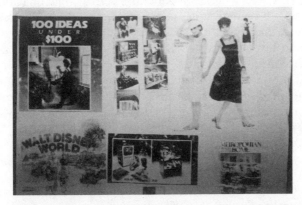

Figure 136. Early in treatment Hispanic chronic patients made collages from magazines.

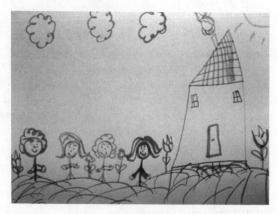

Figure 137. Reunification of her family was a goal for Hispanic Ileana.

own needs aside in serving their families, the group became a place where they could look at and share their own needs, a place and a time where they could do something for themselves.

Termination

Throughout the five months of the group's life, the members' pictures related minimally to their lives in this country despite the fact that most had lived in the United States 10–15 years. Although themes and issues remained relatively constant, there was significant development on the part of some of the participants. For example, when Nora first entered the group, she was very withdrawn with little verbal communication. She did not know how to read or write, had never attended school, and her drawings were pale and small. As the group developed, so did Nora's ability to communicate through her art. By the time it ended, she had come to express her concerns and find joy in her accomplishments. Figure 101 is her bold depiction in red of palm trees, flowers, a chicken, and herself.

The group had been planned for a five-month period, its ending coinciding with Gilda's graduation. As ending drew near, the women who composed it expressed their satisfaction in their drawings. They were proud to show their pictures and they ensured that all who wished had opportunity to discuss their pictures. The spontaneous image-making had provided a vehicle for them to express feelings about the losses they had experienced in leaving their homelands and to give and receive support from one another around this shared experience.

Art Therapy for Acculturation Problems

Immigrants to this country often find themselves strangers in a strange land even years after their migration. Particularly disadvantaged are those with low educational and economic resources. The spontaneous image-making of art therapy can tap the feelings associated with acculturation difficulties. A group setting for this activity is especially beneficial in undercutting the isolation of these individuals. Of particular importance is a therapist sensitive to the culture from which the clients have come.

PSYCHOSOCIAL REHABILITATION

Treatment for chronic post-hospitalization psychiatric patients who have not become integrated into the community is provided through psychosocial rehabilitation services, often utilizing a "clubhouse" model. The goals are oriented toward behavioral changes that will enable the client to learn to function in the community and develop satisfying social relationships. Some centers provide occupational training. There is an emphasis on practical skills and taking responsibility with the "members" of the "clubhouse" encouraged to do much of the activity planning. A non-hierarchical relationship among staff and clientel is fostered with most activity occurring in a group format.

Joanne Ramseyer interned in such a setting during her art therapy master's degree training. The art therapy program she established augmented the facility's goals and in addition provided possibilities beyond other aspects of the program. Particularly in areas of self-awareness, insight, self-disclosure, and the development of creativity and inner resources art therapy was a useful addition to the program. Other goals pursued in the art therapy were anxiety management, increasing self-esteem, problem-solving, and socialization. Most of the work occurred in groups, so interpersonal interaction and engagement with the total program were important aspects of art therapy as well.

Beginning Art Therapy

Del, a man in his mid-20s who was diagnosed manic-depressive with paranoid traits, was attending college when his psychotic symptoms first appeared. He was a highly intelligent individual, acutely aware of his impaired functioning due to his psychiatric disorder. Del was a member of Joanne's art therapy group for nine months. In the early months of his participation he remained aloof from the other group members and be-

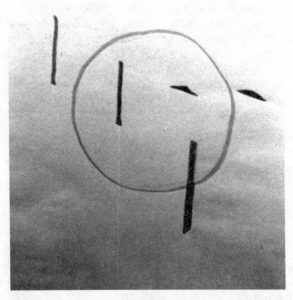

Figure 138. Del was unhappy with his "rigid, controlled" first picture.

came enraged if anyone offered feedback about his art. He was extremely self-critical about his "lack of spontaneity" and described his first picture in art therapy as "disgusting because it was so well-planned and controlled" (Figure 138). Later in therapy he associated his "rigid, disciplined, controlled nature" with his Oriental heritage, particularly his Japanese father. Joanne focussed on ways to teach him to loosen up in his art work and to explore his creations autonomously.

Midphase

Del spent many months experimenting with various media and eventually began to trust Joanne, expressing positive feelings about art therapy to his case worker. She recommended individual art therapy for him in addition to the group. During the three months of his individual sessions, Del explored the content of his drawings much more freely with Joanne.

Of particular importance was his expression of feelings about his family and his mental illness. In Figure 139, he depicted himself in the center with his manic-depressive mother as the circular shape behind him. His

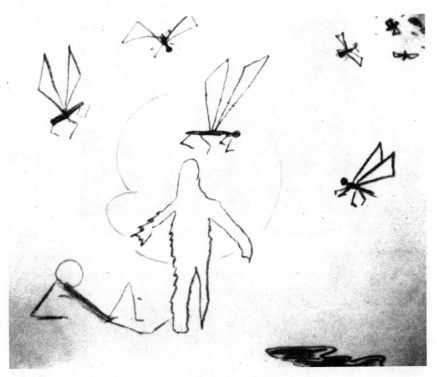

Figure 139. Del's family and mental illness.

brother, also diagnosed manic-depressive, is the stick figure chained to Del's leg on the left. His father is the puddle, lower right, "too strict, rigid, and disinterested in the family to be of any help." Del said he was worn out from being his mother's caretaker and that he feared having to take care of his sick brother as well. He was angry that he himself was sick and no one took care of him. The insects are his "mental illness infiltrating my life."

Joanne asked Del what part of the picture was most important to him and suggested that he elaborate upon it in a second picture. He chose the insects and in Figure 140 drew them inside his head "eating away my brain" and (lower left) throughout his body causing him to jump off a building and lie in a pool of blood (lower center). At lower right is his empty dead body with the insects/illness gone. Del expressed sadness and frustration that no one understood how much he suffered from his condition.

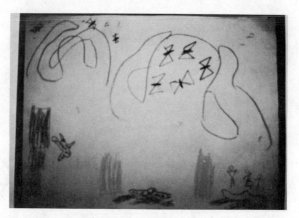

Figure 140. Del being destroyed by his mental illness.

Del continued to attend group art therapy where he made pictures of his feelings of depression and gradually began to share some of his feelings with the others. In individual sessions he spoke of his fear of deteriorating like his mother and his anger towards his father.

Del got in touch with his anger in Figure 141 which shows his Oriental father. Following this, he spent weeks making abstract paintings of his rage. He stated that art therapy was good for him because it countered his tendency to intellectualize and distance himself from his feelings. He started doing art work at home to expand his use of the art therapy

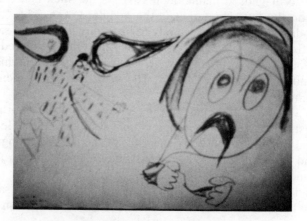

Figure 141. Del's anger at his Oriental father.

process. Evidently, he got a lot out of the ventilation of feelings he was experiencing.

With Joanne's support, Del eventually came to value his intellect and the uniqueness of his art. He became more accepting of his psychiatric condition and stopped blaming himself for his mental illness. His art work reflected the greater freedom he was giving himself as shown in Figure 142.

Termination

As the group was coming to an end, Del said art therapy had been a "welcome relief from talk, talk, talk groups" in which he remained distant from his feelings and others. He continued creating art at home.

It was not customary for the staff of the facility to encourage focus on termination issues, so there was little discussion of ending per se in the art

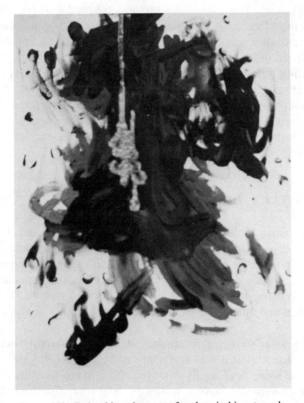

Figure 142. Del achieved greater freedom in his art work.

therapy group. Instead, Joanne planned with the group to have a final art exhibit to which they could invite their family and friends as well as the staff. Much of the energy of the group's final sessions went into planning this event. The show was a great success. Many of the members spoke more of their pictures during this occasion than previously. Seeing them displayed throughout the facility's elegant Victorian house and experiencing the validation of others for their efforts seemed a very positive ending. I attended the exhibit and witnessed the enthusiasm of the members about their art. Many expressed to me how much they would miss Joanne and asked when I would send them another intern so that art therapy could resume. Del gave Joanne a gift, a sculpture he had made from a family portrait he had drawn in art therapy.

Results of Art Therapy Treatment

Del began group art therapy extremely self-critical, untrusting, and isolated from others. The art-making process coupled with sensitive individual art therapy treatment enabled him to explore his painful feelings and to build trust with another. He came to a new self-acceptance, and his final gift to Joanne appeared to be his way of showing appreciation for finally feeling understood. In Del's case, art therapy provided a depth of work not always found in the psychosocial clubhouse model of rehabilitation. Although art therapy in a psychosocial rehabilitation setting is more likely to emphasize socialization, problem-solving, and practical living skills, for some clients it can provide the added balance of intrapsychic processing that they may need.

RESIDENTIAL CARE FOR THE ELDERLY

Like psychosocial rehabilitation, work with the elderly aims for improvement in quality of life rather than emphasizing psychodynamic processes. But unlike psychosocial rehabilitation, the effort is not directed toward integration of the elderly into the community, as the expectation is that nursing home residents will remain there for the rest of their lives. An additional major difference is the functional abilities of the two populations.

In her master's degree internship at a skilled nursing home, Cherie Natenberg found that it was necessary to be resourceful and inventive in enabling the more profoundly disabled residents to use the art materials. Bette, an 83-year-old stroke victim with severe disabling arthritis and impaired hearing, is a case in point.

Beginning Treatment

As with the other residents with whom she worked, Cherie's goals for Bette's art therapy were social and emotional growth, raised self-esteem, and rehabilitation of physical problems through manipulation of the media. In Bette's case, the latter goal augmented the former ones.

Bette was confined to a wheelchair. She had use of neither hand, both of which were contracted into fists from arthritis. Arthritis affected her neck as well causing her head to face down most of the time. She had difficulties speaking so that her words came out very slowly and with much effort. She wore a hearing-aid. Bette had suffered from arthritis since childhood and at the time she began art therapy, participated in no activities. She had been in a nursing home for 23 years. As a younger woman, however, she was an accomplished artist. Bette's only family was a sister with whom she was very close. The sister called her every day and visited frequently.

Cherie devised a Velcro® strap for Bette to enable her to hold a paint brush. Although Bette was right-handed, Cherie wrapped it around her stronger left hand and wedged the brush into it (see Figure 15). After several sessions, Bette developed very good control in using it. Cherie also arranged several colors of paints in a flat dish and provided water in a low bowl so that Bette could dip her brush into them easily. In this way, Bette could paint for the first time in many years.

Bette participated in an art therapy group with three other women whose physical impairment was so severe that they could not take care of their personal needs. Cognitive impairment for the four women, however, was very slight. Nevertheless, they were quite concrete and abstract thinking was difficult for them. Their concerns were the problems of everyday living. In her work with them, Cherie sought to help them maintain the defenses necessary to function optimally in the institution, recognizing that they would likely not improve physically or return home. There was extensive drawing and painting, but little insight-oriented discussion of the art. Cherie tried to provide an opportunity for the expression of feeling through art, social interaction around the activity, and a focus on the here-and-now issues they expressed.

Midphase

Four months into art therapy, Cherie suggested that the group "draw a wish." Figure 143 is Bette's rendition. She usually portrayed happy subjects that protected her from any confrontive issues. In this session she painted slowly, stretching out the activity as long as possible. She painted

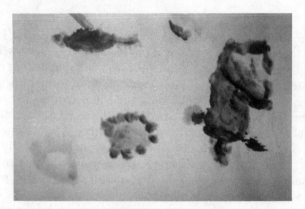

Figure 143. Elderly Bette's wish for good food.

bread, lobster, chicken, and steak, saying that her wish was for a "decent meal." Meal times were significant events at the nursing home, providing the elderly with an important source of pleasure. As was illustrated in the early work of dually diagnosed Dobie, nourishment in the concrete form of food is a common symbol of needs.

Cherie began seeing Bette in individual sessions as well. Two months later in an individual session, Bette drew a wish again, Figure 144. The picture shows a waterfall, children around a campfire, and the water flowing out to the ocean. Bette said that her wish was to swim again as she had before her arthritis became severe. For the first time, she acknowledged her disease and said that she felt terrible about being so disabled but didn't want to talk about it yet. This picture not only illustrates Bette's emotional progress in individual art therapy, but also shows her increased investment in her art and the control and skill she had developed in using the Velcro strap to hold the paint brush.

There were other changes as well. Bette's attitude and appearance improved. She began wearing makeup and going to the hairdresser at the home. She talked more frequently and with less strain. She looked forward to art therapy. Bette's sister called Cherie frequently to comment on Bette's improvement. Six months after beginning art therapy, Bette picked up a paint brush and began painting before Cherie had time to attach the Velcro devise to her hand. She never used it again.

Termination

There was a possibility that Cherie would be hired by the nursing home following graduation, in which case her work with Bette would continue.

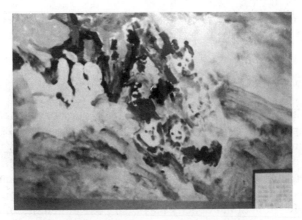

Figure 144. Bette's wish to be able to swim again.

This sort of uncertainty often clouds the termination process in work of graduating interns. As it turned out, Cherie chose to take a position elsewhere. Bette and her sister expressed much appreciation to Cherie and the sister brought her a corsage for a goodbye celebration. Cherie had become very fond of Bette and had derived a great deal of gratification from the changes art therapy had wrought in this severely impaired woman. From time to time after her departure, Cherie visited her at the home. Approximately one year later Bette died. Tribute was paid to Cherie at the funeral for the importance of her work in adding to the quality of Bette's final years.

Results of Treatment

A combination of physical rehabilitation and a caring relationship fostered first physical activity then increased imagistic expressiveness for this severely impaired woman. Most consequential was the effect this progression had upon her life outside art therapy. For Bette there was improved self-esteem, increased communication with others, and a more positive outlook on life.

Art Therapy With the Elderly

As dramatized in the work with Bette, art therapy can fulfill a variety of needs for the elderly. Physical impairment characteristic of residents of nursing homes requires sensitivity and inventiveness on the part of the art therapist in facilitating use of art materials. The possibilities for self-expression and relationship that art therapy affords can have a significant impact on nursing home residents whose lives may have become quite limited and circumscribed.

CONCLUSION

The preceding examples illustrate work with populations other than in the traditional psychiatric settings where most art therapists work. The varying needs and conditions of these clients point up the necessity for flexibility and resourcefulness on the part of the art therapist.

For some populations, language deficits may prove a communication barrier as is the case for some who are dually diagnosed, immigrants, and some elderly. Functional deficits may also pose difficulties in both intellectual and physical realms as illustrated by the dually diagnosed and some of the elderly. Societal integration is a concern in psychosocial rehabilitation and those incarcerated for crimes.

Despite the large differences in population, conditions of treatment, length of therapy, and treatment goals, attributes of treatment phase remain relatively universal. Assessment, development of treatment goals, and engagement characterize the beginning phase. There may be significant differences in how engagement is achieved, however. For example, in beginning work with dually diagnosed Tommy, it was necessary for Ellen Sontag to limit his choice of art materials to media that would not induce chaotic regression. Rose Marano Geiser created a receptive atmosphere for jailed Terry to ventilate about her crime of murdering her daughter. Cherie Natenberg devised a Velcro strap to enable arthritis-ridden Bette to hold a paint brush.

For all the clients, mid-phase was a period of getting down to serious therapeutic work after having established an engagement in art therapy. Gilda Moreno's Hispanic group of chronic patients shared images of their continued attachment to their lost countries of origin. Del, Joanne Ramsayer's client in psychosocial rehabilitation, worked through his harsh self-critical views and found expression of his rage through his art. Del and incarcerated Terry explored family relationships. Dually diagnosed Tommy and Dobie dealt with loss of family. Elderly and impaired Bette transferred her accomplishments in art to a more positive outlook in other areas.

Termination was the most varied of the stages. As discussed in Chapter 8, the circumstances of termination differ widely. Most of the terminations illustrated here resulted from the ending of the art therapist's assignment to the treatment facility, a common occurrence at training sites. In addition to this arbitrary determination of an ending date are the difficult feelings attending separation. Nevertheless, in most examples presented here, length of treatment was determined in advance, therefore the therapy was planned accordingly. There were some unexpected outcomes, however. Although the psychosocial rehabilitation facility at which Joanne Ramsayer interned discouraged a focus on termination, her clients there chose to make use of their final art exhibit for some of the taking-stock and saying good-bye process of termination. A frequent possibility in many facilities is the sudden transfer or discharge of a patient such as Rose Marano Geiser experienced in her work at the jail. In Terry's treatment there had been much termination work, but the final leave-taking was aborted. On the other hand, a well-planned termination phase can help the client to integrate previous losses, as in the case of dually diagnosed Dobie.

Finally, the variety of work presented in this chapter to illustrate the diversity of the stages of treatment in different settings may raise the question, "Does all of this constitute art psychotherapy?" The importance of the context of art therapy in determining its nature is the subject of the next section. Chapter 12 focuses specifically on the question of "art psychotherapy" and "art as therapy."

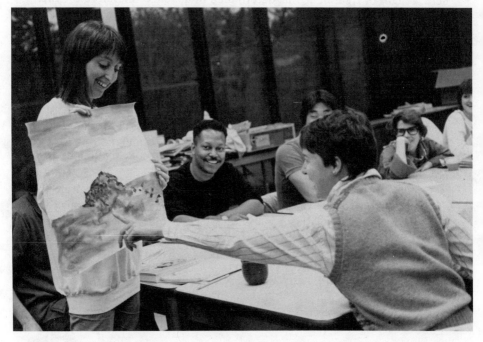

Figure 145. Relating to art expressions often generates animated discussion in art therapy classes. Here, student Mary Cairns points to picture art therapy teacher Pat Allen is holding.

PART FOUR

Context of Art Therapy

The framework surrounding art therapy treatment, from the immediate structure of the treatment facility to the prevailing social attitudes and values of the culture in which it is embedded, compose the background for the work. Background influences are often so taken for granted that their enormous impact is overlooked.

Chapter 10 focuses on the social forces that shape art therapy, and Chapter 11 delineates some of the power dynamics of the politics of art therapy to which they give rise. A background influence unique to art therapy is art therapists' historical heritage of a polarity within the field, often designated as the "art as therapy" and "art psychotherapy" dichotomy. Chapter 12 addresses this often muddied muddle.

Art therapy training has developed to prepare students to practice in settings where art therapists usually work. In this way, it too is greatly influenced by context. The preparation of an art therapist requires intense, demanding comprehensive work. Although Chapter 13 outlines the basic ingredients of that training, it focuses more on its unique processes and their desired outcomes. There is a special emphasis on the enhancement of awareness through art expression and the use of creativity in education. A discussion of advanced training looks to future needs and developments in the profession.

The final chapter of the book looks to the potential of the art therapy process for wholeness and spiritual healing. A framework for understanding art therapy processing in a larger than psychotherapeutic context is offered with examples of imagery evoked by existential questing.

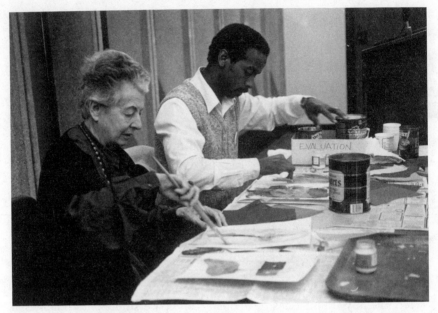

Figure 146. Edith Wallace conducting a workshop on active imagination accompanied by art therapy student Tony Porter.

CHAPTER 10

Social Forces

Art therapists work within a constellation of interlocking matrices. Discussions of art therapy practice often neglect the powerful influences of the many layers of atmosphere that surround and bear upon the work at hand. In an account of an art therapy session or case, we usually hear what the patient did and said, perhaps the interaction between therapist and patient, and the patient's background, but seldom the subtle framework in which the work is embedded.

Figure 147, composed of rectangles representing structured systems and circles representing communities, is a simplified diagram of matrices in which any one art therapist's work resides. Usually she works in a unit or department in a facility which is a part of a larger system. That system has a place in its own geographical context (neighborhood, city, county, state), as well as in the larger society as a part of an overall service system (such as the structuring of mental health or educational services in this country). Finally, all of the aforementioned exist within a highly complex amorphous, diverse, and sometimes contradictory belief and value system. This culture is shaped by prevailing attitudes and definitions regarding mental health, human understanding and growth, education, art, and the other goals that are a part of the art therapist's work.

Additionally the art therapist has a place within her profession, and art therapy has a place in larger systems of the professional community. I will discuss these various matrices beginning with the smaller, more particular units and their subsystems, then moving to the larger, less clear realms. Please bear in mind that I am not attempting a thorough sociometric analysis, but only a brief view in order to enlarge awareness of the influence of these systems and subsystems on the art therapist's work.

TREATMENT FACILITY

Most art therapists work within an institution such as a hospital, school, or clinic. Naturally the type, size, mission, and philosophy of the institution have a strong influence on the work. For example, art therapy in a

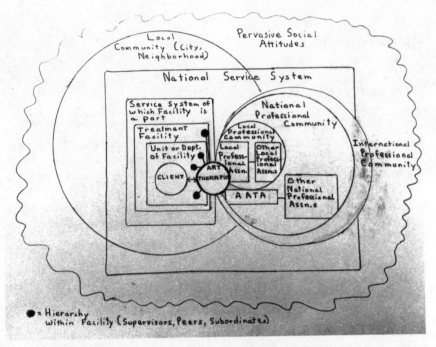

Figure 147. A diagram of the matrices in which an art therapist works.

school for emotionally disturbed children would be very different from art therapy on a short-term hospital unit for psychotic patients. Further, if the institution uses a psychoanalytic orientation, for example, art therapy would be expected to follow that philosophical approach compared to a facility that relies on behavior modification for treatment. So before an art therapist is even hired, much has already been determined about the nature of her work.

The subsystem of the facility is the unit or department in which the art therapist works. It may be a hospital ward or an expressive or activity therapy department which services a number of wards. A small clinic may not be divided into departments, and the art therapist may be simply a part of the staff. In any case, she has a position on the hierarchal ladder. All too often it is closer to the bottom than to the top. In hospitals, usually Doctors of Medicine are in positions of clinical authority. In schools the principal is the director. Positions of lesser authority are held by other doctors in hospitals and other educators in schools. Even though the art therapist may have no wish to have administrative authority, administrative positions are often the only route to high status in a facility. Art therapists often hold "adjunctive" positions as part of a treatment team. Unfortunately their abilities, expertise, and contributions may be relegated to an "adjunctive" position as well. This problem was raised in connection with the art therapist's identity in Chapter 1 and will be discussed further in Chapter 11. For now, we will examine the overview of the total matrix in order to see its interactional systems.

Unless the art therapist is part of an expressive therapies department, her immediate supervisor is likely to be a nonart therapist who may have little understanding of her work. The economics of the facility may be such that third-party payments are not available for art therapists, as opposed to other treatment personnel on the staff, and thereby further limit the work, the value it is given, and the salary of the art therapist.

In addition to the formal hierarchy, the informal chain of command should not be underestimated. For example, at one time my place in a hospital hierarchy was considered by a ward administrator to be higher than some of the junior psychiatrists because I was writing a paper with the section chief. At another time a research assistant had considerable power because she and the project director were secretly engaged to be married. I have known of instances where art therapy was established with some reservations, yet the art therapist "proved" herself and the value of her contribution so that she eventually attained a position of high respect.

A more distant and sometimes less apparent influence is the larger system in which the treatment facility resides. It might be a county school system or a hospital program operated by a management firm or organization of which the hospital is a part (e.g., the Veteran's Administration). The Clinical Center of the NIH where I worked for many years was a part of the Department of Health, Education, and Welfare of the Federal Government. Often the larger system determines such issues as pay scale and the mission of the facility. Unfortunately, economic considerations provide the major impetus in many policy determinations. More about that in the next chapter.

PROFESSIONAL COMMUNITY

The art therapist may be more or less involved in the professional community of which she is a part. Nevertheless, the professional community exerts a strong influence on her work. Her training was obtained through some resource within the professional community. She may pursue continuing education in the form of workshops, courses, and conferences. She may have art therapy colleagues or receive supervision from an art therapist outside her facility. She may also have colleagues or supervisors from other disciplines. The professional community extends through matrices of the local community, the national professional community, and the international professional community. Whether the art therapist has any contact with other professionals or not, the development of the profession of art therapy within the matrix of the other mental health and educational professions influences her work.

The art therapist may be a part of a local art therapy association or the profession's national organization, the American Art Therapy Association. In any case, organized art therapy has done much to put art therapy on the map, through publications, conferences, lobbying, and the like. Any individual art therapist's work is influenced by the perception others have of the field, whether they be clients or the administrators who hire her or the colleagues from other disciplines who refer her clients. The perceptions of art therapy carried by these people are often strongly influenced by the efforts of organized art therapy to make the profession known.

The field has continued to advance in its sophistication, training standards, credentialing, and so forth, largely as the result of efforts by organized art therapy. In some instances the professional association has worked with other professional associations to advance understanding of art therapy. Individuals work through art therapy associations as well as through their own systems to advance the profession. As an art therapy educator, I feel it is my responsibility to elevate the field as much as I am able by screening candidates for admission and by providing the best training possible. As a relatively new profession, art therapy continues to suffer lack of recognition of its potential in some quarters.

NATIONAL SERVICE SYSTEM

All of these influences are embedded in a national service delivery system. It is a system of hospitals, schools, clinics, homes for the elderly, neighborhood centers, prisons, and so forth, both in the private and public sector. We take for granted the institutions through which we try to provide healing and growth. That we structure such experiences in the forms that we do determines the nature of their delivery. For example, in our culture hospitalization on a psychiatric unit for one who believes himself possessed by evil spirits is a very different method and experience from a visit with the medicine man, which may be the appropriate treatment in another culture. It is important that those in service capacities, including art therapists, be cognizant of the limitations these systems impose, with a view to their improvement and in some instances the possibility for development of alternative systems. For example, an art therapy student recently completed an independent study project in which she created a model for a holistic health center where the arts play a major part in treatment.

LOCAL COMMUNITY

In addition to being a part of the professional matrix, the art therapist's facility is also part of the local community. Treatment in a small rural area where everyone knows everyone else may be different from that in a large city. A facility in an affluent suburb may be under pressures and influences that differ from that in an inner-city ghetto. You will note that in the diagram in Figure 147 the facility and the service system in which it resides are located in both the local community and in the national service system. They are shown overlapping rather than one being embedded in the other. The local professional community naturally is located in the local community, but also within the national delivery system. The national professional community, on the other hand, is located in the national service system, but not in the local community. (It was a bit difficult to diagram.)

SOCIAL ATTITUDES

Finally, Figure 147 illustrates the pervasive social attitudes as an amorphous, indefinite mass in which the entire system resides. This mass is unclear, subject to much variety, and is even contradictory in some areas. It is a fluctuating field that changes continuously. For example, when I first entered the mental health field in the early 1960s, "broken homes" were considered a source of developmental trouble for the "unfortunate" children they spawned. Today, the term "broken homes" is hardly ever heard. Society has changed and divorce is a common family condition rather than the exceptional casualty. Within the last two decades the issues of minority rights, women's rights, gay rights, rights of the elderly and handicapped point up other areas that have changed in the ways we view ourselves and one another and therefore the ways in which we define mental illness and health and what we do about them.

I was in San Francisco in 1970 for the American Psychiatric Association Annual Conference at which there was a demonstration by gay activists. Subsequently, the *Diagnostic and Statistical Manual of the American Psychiatric Association* eliminated homosexuality from its category of diagnostic syndromes (Edition III). The point is that it was not the mental health professions who were taking the leadership in defining what is considered emotional disturbance, but rather that the professional community was responding to changes in societal attitudes. In the early 1970s, I found Phyllis Chesler's *Women and Madness* (1972) a startling outcry against the mistreatment of women by the mental health professions. Largely as a result of the women's movement, expectations for women have changed considerably since the book's publication. It's not too likely that a woman these days would be considered emotionally unbalanced for wanting more self-fulfillment than marriage and motherhood can provide.

These two examples of homosexuality and women's issues are good examples of both the flux and variety in social attitudes. Most of us have lived long enough to have witnessed and experienced the change in societal viewpoints around these issues. Most of us know people with varying attitudes on these subjects, sometimes accompanied by strong feeling. It is within this milieu that psychological treatment is defined and operationalized.

This chapter has provided an overview of the framework of the interconnections of structures, networks, and the conceptual dispositions that generate them. At each juncture there is political activity that supports, impinges upon, and otherwise shapes the art therapist's work. The next chapter discusses the nature of some of these operations in the politics of art therapy.

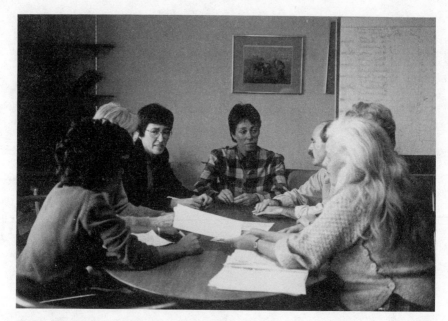

Figure 148. Staff meeting at CAUSES, Child Abuse Unit, Illinois Masonic Hospital, at which author (right) consults on patient art.

CHAPTER 11

Professional Politics

No art therapist works in isolation. Even those in private practice are influenced by the mental health delivery system, the local community, the professional community, and obviously by pervasive social attitudes. Professional politics here refers to the ways individuals and groups interact to operate the system. To discuss all the possible particulars of the framework diagrammed in Figure 147 would take more volumes than I would care to write or you would care to read. I will try to touch only upon those points that I consider most crucial.

WITHIN THE FACILITY

The facility provides the five-days-a-week milieu for most art therapists. It is from the facility that she receives her paycheck. The concretization of her work is in the facility. This is not the place of abstract ideas. This is the grappling place of everyday reality. It is here that she has most problems.

The prime issue is one of power. Where does the art therapist reside in the institution's hierarchy? Recently an art therapy colleague told me how hard it was for her to move from a small clinic where she had worked for many years as a part of the treatment and planning staff to the larger structure of a hospital where she was a member of the adjunctive therapy department, or as she described herself, a "peon."

Position in the Hierarchy

The art therapist's position may be unclear, as mine was when I worked at the NIH. I was attached to a research project, but not to any professional group, such as doctors, nurses, social workers, occupational therapists, aides, research assistants, or secretaries. Those workers knew their places both within their group and in the larger hierarchy. My unclear role caused me much confusion. Early on I felt like a student. Later I felt like a professional. Sometimes I felt like an expert, sometimes like a "peon." One minute I would be asked to appear on the radio on behalf of NIH or have an exhibit I had created represent NIH at its 25th Anniversary celebration. The next minute I would feel not only invisible but inaudible in a staff meeting. One minute my ideas would be discounted by the doctors who were in charge. The next minute they would ask me to provide art therapy for a case that defied other approaches, and then they would rave about how more happened in one art therapy session than in 10 psychiatric sessions. Some nurses and occupational therapists welcomed the richness art therapy added to the milieu. Others were threatened by it.

I worked at NIH during the 1960s and early 1970s. I ended up as the only female non-M.D. member of the unit's research team. During the times I felt discounted, I puzzled as to whether it was because I was not an M.D., because I was "just a woman," or for personal reasons. When another female researcher/clinician (a social worker whom I respected highly) told me she experienced the same thing, I realized that our being women was a significant factor. Clearly there were differences among the relationships with particular staff members as well as with the different units on which I worked. Some were characterized by much mutual respect and warm personal feelings. Others had a chill to them that was often disturbing and sometimes puzzling to me.

I tell students that working with patients is easy; it's the staff that's difficult. Some students have had the exhilirating winds of accomplishment taken from their sails by the resentment they've experienced from staff members. One of our otherwise excellent student placements had to be discontinued because the student was caught in the cross-fire between her art therapist supervisor there and the supervisor's supervisor, an occupational therapist, who wanted to supervise the student as well. The power struggle between the two eventuated in their both leaving the institution.

Supervisor

The question of the art therapist's supervisor is a very significant one. Often it is not another art therapist when there is not one on the staff. We hope it is someone who respects the art therapist's work and recognizes its value to the treatment program. Those who are not art persons themselves may recognize the art therapist's area of expertise and encourage her creativity in maximizing the art therapy contribution to the unit. Less fortunate for the art therapist is the supervisor who feels competent in the art therapy realm and therefore prescribes the art therapist's work. I have heard art therapists complain about occupational therapist supervisors who had art experience in their professional training and therefore viewed art therapy as a specialty of occupational therapy. Although some of the activities in the two fields are similar, the approaches and goals are often vastly different. Furthermore, the lower a person is on the hierarchal totem pole, the less power he or she has and therefore the more power he or she needs, often leading to authoritarian control. Unfortunately, occupational therapy, like art therapy, is sometimes considered a filler of time rather than a crucial treatment modality and as a result at times is accorded little power in the system. In contrast, I have known of many situations, some of them my own experiences, where there were excellent relationships and understanding between occupational therapy and art therapy, including supervisory relationships. Nevertheless, because the boundaries between the two ways of working are easily blurred, I do not put students in practicum placements where they would be supervised by occupational therapists. Students usually have enough confusion and identity problems to work on as it is.

Professional Identity

The identity of the art therapist is discussed in Chapter 1. How she is viewed at her facility is influenced by many factors in an interaction between what she brings to her position, how the position is structured within the facility, and what views of art therapy the other staff may bring to the facility. All these conditions are influenced by all the matrices diagrammed in Figure 147 and discussed previously. Nevertheless, the art therapist's identity is not static. As I mentioned earlier, I began work at the NIH more or less as a student. Although my position remained ambiguous, at the time I left several psychiatrists were fighting over who would get my office. Desirable office space was one of the most obvious emblems of status, and mine was clearly especially attractive.

There is much that the art therapist can do to enhance her value to the treatment program as well as to potentiate opportunities for her creative participation in decisions affecting her work. In the training program I direct, students are expected as a part of their practicum experience to educate other staff about art therapy. This can occur in informal contacts, staff meetings at which the art therapist presents material about particular patients, and at in-service training sessions. Many of my students have developed experiential in-service training workshops for their particular placement sites. These are usually enthusiastically received. Where an experiential session might not be well received, slide presentations and discussion of patient art work are often both informative and stimulating. At one such program I attended that was part of a monthly educational series for the entire mental hospital, we were told that no program previously held had been so well-attended as the art therapy presentation.

Even more fundamental than the specific educational opportunities the art therapist may develop for her facility is her basic attitude toward her work and toward her own competency. In a facility run by more seasoned professionals from more established professions, it may be difficult for the art therapist to recognize herself as an expert. If her training has been thorough (see Chapter 13 for discussion of training) and she continues to advance her learning beyond her formal education, she should be competent in understanding and performing psychotherapy. Beyond that, she has an expertise in art therapy that nonart therapy staff members do not possess. No one is more qualified than she to develop an art therapy treatment program, to encourage and understand patient art therapy, and to relate to clientele around art in therapy. All too often, however, art therapists are intimidated by more established professionals, especially since they occupy rungs higher on the hierarchal ladder. The art therapist's low paycheck may reinforce her feelings of limited power and competency within the system. Nevertheless, there are many art therapists I know who started out in relatively low level or questionable positions but established themselves as highly respected and integral members of the facility's treatment staff.

When I first started working at the NIH Clinical Center, the ward clerk would make dentist and X-ray appointments for patients during times they were scheduled to see me; doctors would barge into art therapy sessions to summon patients for unscheduled appointments; and nurses would tease patients about their art. During the early 1960s, few had heard of art therapy and it was not taken seriously. It was not long, however, before staff became familiar with my work through staff meetings and in-service workshops I organized, and the disruptive interference soon ceased.

Another clash in my experience occurred when I entered graduate school for an M.S.W. degree after over a decade of art therapy practice and research. At my field work placement I attempted to introduce art therapy. I broached the subject to my social worker supervisor who was familiar with my work and supportive of my suggestion. She took my request to the psychologist who was clinical director. She reported that he was not interested in making art therapy a part of the facility's program. I was to be content with using it where appropriate with individual clients or as a small part of the two groups I was coleading. Staff meetings consisted of lectures from the consulting psychiatrist who screened all admissions so I had no opportunity to present my work there, and I did not want to go over my supervisor's head by speaking with the clinical director myself. Clearly he considered me merely a student.

The facility was involved in a research project at a nearby university. My supervisor suggested that I involve myself in it by presenting art therapy to the research group there. I did and was invited to serve as a consultant as a part of my field work until graduation and continue for the usual consultant's fee thereafter.

The contrast in my position at the two institutions was extreme. At the agency I was treated as a student with much to learn and little to contribute beyond client care. At the research project I was an expert expected to develop a research design, and I was given resources, space, time, and clients to carry it through.

Toward the end of my field work, students were invited to present their work at an agency staff meeting. I showed examples of art therapy. The clinical director became excited, gave me funds to buy art supplies, and urged me to develop as much art therapy as I could before I graduated. It was too little too late. He had seen me as a student, which I was, rather than as an experienced professional with art therapy's unique expertise, which I was also.

I recently spoke with the principal of a school for emotionally disturbed children who asked me to recommend an art therapist for a part-time position. She said that there was a half-hour in the adolescents' class schedule she would like to fill with art therapy. I explained that 30 minutes is too short a time period for an adolescent group to orient itself, make art, process it, and clean up. The point is that an art therapist can better assess the art therapy needs and appropriate structure for a particular population than other staff. Sometimes art therapists are required by administrators to see patients in larger groups than are effective. It is important for the art therapist to assert herself regarding art therapy planning. The school principal wanted to hire an art therapist for an untenable position.

Sometimes even more touchy than scheduling is interpretation of patient art. I have always tried to encourage staff to respond to the art in order to involve them further in art therapy rather than to act as though it is a mysterious realm accessible only to the initiated. Nevertheless, if I feel art products are being over-interpreted, misread, disrespected, or not taken seriously, I attempt to provide gentle guidance. I have seldom encountered problems in this area. People are generally not so confident of their own reactions to art to be closed to another way of looking at it.

Interestingly, such problems are more likely to occur between two art therapists. With others, however, it is the art therapist's responsibility to provide education in understanding the art as well as in the other aspects of the work. Usually this is easily accomplished through example. When the art therapist brings the art to a staff meeting and discusses the session and the art, others glean the method of the art therapist's understanding.

At the other extreme from being given too little respect, sometimes art therapy is considered almost magical in its potency and the art therapist something of a divinator. Chapter 7 discusses the pressure sometimes brought to bear on the art therapist to use the art for formulation of a definitive diagnosis. Where such a diagnosis is not possible, it is necessary for the art therapist to point up the limitations of the work, as well as its benefits. Usually there is significant information that comes from an art therapy session, even if not a complete diagnosis.

Facility's Approach and Methods

An art therapy student took a summer position at a camp for emotionally disturbed children. She returned disappointed, frustrated with the camp's rigid behavior modification program that contradicted the more dynamic approach to clients she had been taught. Another student was offered a job at a school for the emotionally disturbed that also operated on a behavior modification model with an elaborate system of rewards and punishments. Needing the job, the student took on the challenge of trying to integrate a dynamic and humanistic art therapy tradition into a behavior modification framework.

The question raised by these two examples is how the art therapist relates to the overall mission, philosophy, and practice of the facility in which she works. One of the things I loved about working at NIH was that all treatment was absolutely free. No patient was ever turned away for lack of finances or discharged because insurance had been used up. On the other hand, there were times I felt that patients were treated as research subjects (which they were), rather than as human beings (which they were also).

Many art therapists are frustrated in working on short-term units where there is insufficient time to develop a meaningful relationship with the patient. Recidivism is often high, and the art therapist may wonder if the patient benefits from the brief treatment program at all. Most art therapists cannot afford the luxury of being "choicy" (as an elderly woman from the rural South used to say) in selecting their jobs. Some graduates have complained that they were overskilled for the menial chores that some art therapists are required to perform.

So what is an art therapist to do under these less than perfect conditions? At NIH I spoke up when I felt patients were not being treated properly. This was not always easy. One ward administrator gave me the dubious title of the ward's "gadfly for patient rights."

I believe it is the art therapist's responsibility, as it is every other staff member's responsibility, to ensure the facility's functioning for the greatest benefit of its clientele. Staff members' active acceptance of this responsibility, both individually and collectively can have a significant impact. On the other hand, I do not expect an art therapist to remake the world, or even the system in which she works. Often there are severe economic limitations. Sometimes the art therapist is faced with the difficult choice of remaining at a facility where she cannot support the treatment philosophy or methods or taking her chances elsewhere. Art therapy is still a young profession with fewer positions than practitioners, so giving up an art therapy position may be a considerable sacrifice. Nevertheless, a responsible art therapist will weigh all the factors involved in making such a decision. She will view her own work and the facility's work critically. She will consider what needs to be changed, how that can be effected, and what part she can play. She will recognize what cannot be changed and her own limitations in effecting change. In other words, she will not simply be a passive cog in the facility's machinery. The human service field demands informed and active participation in this direction.

PROFESSIONAL COMMUNITY

Whereas the art therapist usually works in a hierarchal system with a more or less clear chain of command at her facility, her relationships within the professional community are likely to be more informal and diverse. In discussing the professional community I will begin with art therapy, including organized art therapy, and then proceed to the larger mental health and educational communities.

Art Therapy

If the art therapist is active in either her local professional organization (e.g., the Illinois Art Therapy Association if she lives in Chicago) or the national professional society (the American Art Therapy Association) then she plays in the political games that characterize such organizations. She may be a part of a faction united by philosophical approach, educational background, or personal affinity. She may hold office or work on a

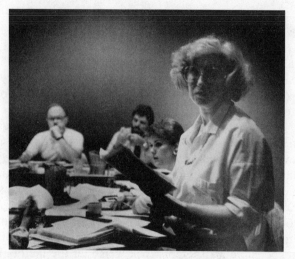

Figure 149. Helen Landgarten, treasurer, presents the budget report at an American Art Therapy Association Executive Board Meeting.

committee. In spite of their sometimes tiresome political machinations, these organizations are of enormous benefit to the profession as well as to the individual art therapist. As is obvious, art therapists can develop the profession collectively far more effectively and efficiently than would be possible singly. In the relatively brief period since its establishment in 1969, the American Art Therapy Association has enabled the profession to make impressive strides in the recognition and respect accorded art therapy, in training of art therapists, in scholarly publications and conferences, in communication both within the profession and with allied professions, and in lobbying. For an art therapist who works in isolation from other art therapists, the professional association can provide a support system and forum for the exchange of ideas. Much less frequently art therapists join together informally in study groups or other gatherings to exchange ideas.

As in other fields, art therapy has its systems of seniority, reigning dignitaries, and the like. These social and political realities play a part in the individual art therapist's work as she may try to advance herself within the profession through publishing, presenting at conferences, working on committees, or running for office in professional societies. These distinctions may or may not enhance her status at the facility where she works.

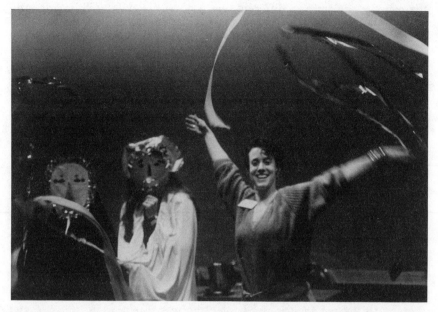

Figure 150. AATA Annual Conferences provide opportunities for participation in creative workshops such as "Uncovering Our Outer Mask," here conducted by Elizabeth Spear Rogers (right).

Allied Professions

Usually, the art therapist works with other professionals such as doctors, nurses, psychologists, social workers, occupational, recreational, expressive therapists, educators, and so forth. In a parallel manner, art therapy takes it place among the other allied professions. The individual art therapist is both influenced by this relationship and influences it. For example, the art therapy profession as a whole does not enjoy the status of psychiatry. The individual art therapist is regarded in this context. On the other hand, should her particular work be recognized as impressive, those who see it as such are likely to increase their respect for the profession as a whole.

Art therapists want the respect of other professionals who are in positions to hire or promote them. I write this having just chaired a panel discussion on art therapy research. Panelists were saying that "we need to speak the language of the other professions"; "research will validate the profession and gain us third-party payments"; and so forth. I agree that these are valuable goals, but I see the route toward the destination the panelists desire as a different one. I don't believe it will be primarily by speaking a language that we did nor evolve nor by doing research in the manner of physical or social sciences that we will receive respect (although such language access may increase communication and such research might contribute to the general body of knowledge). In my experience, respect for art therapy has evolved through personal contact. A clinical director to whose program an art therapist has made an impressive contribution will want to hire art therapists in the future. In fact, I had one such experience in establishing our master's degree program at the University of Illinois/Chicago. I was trying to set up a practicum placement at a prestigious teaching hospital in Chicago. After many delays from an apparently disinterested staff, I was finally invited for a visit to look at the facility and tell the staff about our program. I wasn't particularly optimistic because so many roadblocks had been thrown in the way previously. At the meetings with the staff, the clinical director made an unexpected appearance, because he had just heard of the nature of the meeting. Previously he had been on the psychiatric staff of the Menninger Foundation where he was familiar with the art therapy work of Robert Ault there. As a result, he was most enthusiastic about our bringing art therapy to the psychiatric department he was directing in Chicago, and that placement developed into a fine learning experience for our students. Apparently the students carried on the tradition of providing a significant service, because when we did not place a student at the hospital for one of our rotations, the psychiatric supervisor there was quite upset. It was clear that they valued the art therapy contribution highly.

As to research contributions, I do not disagree with the many art therapy leaders who wish to encourage art therapy research to promote the status of the profession. I do see the picture differently from those who wish to tailor art therapy research designs to fit the existing methodologies of the physical and behavioral sciences, however. So often, quantifying art data is reductionistic to the point of destroying its meaningfulness. There is need for art therapists to develop our own methodologies that better suit our form of data so that the art may be viewed more holistically. In my experience, those of the allied professions have been open to such possibilities. Their interests have been that I produce research, not how it is accomplished. An example was the chief of a prestigious hospital's psychiatric service who wanted me to head his large activities department in order to gain, as he put it, another research investigator in addition to the slots he already had for that purpose. He saw me as able to wear three hats: art therapist, administrator, and researcher.

The point is that it is art therapists themselves who limit art therapy research to a reductionistic treatment of the data, not pressures exerted from those outside the field. It is art therapists who believe art therapists must "speak the language" of more prestigious disciplines. In my experience, nonart therapy researchers have been excited by the art data and interested in finding new ways to work with it.

The inequities in status among mental health professions often lead to differential pay scales among clinicians performing the same or comparable work. All might be psychotherapists with the same responsibilities and competence, yet the psychiatrist is likely to be paid most, the psychologist next, then the social worker. The art therapist's work is different but comparable, sometimes more competent, sometimes less. Yet in general, her pay is likely to be less. It is in this way and others that the art therapist is influenced by the larger system of the mental health community. She may depend on its nonart therapy members for referral if she wishes to have a private practice. Because of these inequities, some art therapists have obtained additional credentials in order to pass through doors not open to them as art therapists. I obtained a Master of Social Work degree in order to collect third-party payment for my already-established private practice (possible in Maryland where I began my practice) and a Ph.D. in order to teach art therapy at a university.

Taken to an extreme, a trend such as this could lead to art therapy becoming a subspecialty of the more established professions of social work and clinical psychology. Each year, I hear of more and more people with a master's degree in art therapy (the terminal degree in the field) pursuing another master's degree or a Ph.D. (This issue is discussed from a different angle in Chapter 13.) The core of art therapy is imagistic expression, requiring of the practitioner much more than a superficial acquaintance with art. Therefore, it is not likely that other mental health professionals who have not made a sizeable emotional commitment to their own art-making will become more than dabblers in art therapy techniques. It would be unfortunate indeed if art therapy lost its dynamism by merging with other professions in such a way as to dilute its potency.

The inequities among the professions lead to consequential results for art therapists. They must often depend on professionals in more established fields for referrals and hiring. Organized art therapy has made many efforts to demonstrate to psychiatrists and other mental health administrators the effectiveness of art therapy through presentations and publications aimed especially for them. There have been instances where professionals with higher status and fees have exploited professionals of lower status and fees. Both in private practice and in hospitals I have known of groups co-led by a psychiatrist and a social worker, nurse, or art therapist where the patient paid psychiatric rates of which the psychiatrist's cotherapist received only a small fraction. In one hospital group of which I was aware, the psychiatrist at times didn't even attend some of the group meetings.

If these aspects of the politics of art therapy seem rather dismal, bear in mind that there have been impressive strides made in areas such as civil service classification, particularly on the part of organized art therapy. The field placements of training programs have introduced art therapy in many facilities with the result that art therapy positions are now a regular part of the staff make-up in increasing numbers of facilities. Further, organized art therapy is working toward licensing and eventual third-party payment. The increasingly high caliber of art therapy that has re-sulted from the continuing development of the field through improvement in training, growth in sophistication in professional publications, and pro-fessional maturity of organized art therapy all contribute to the general elevation of the profession.

On the other side of the equation is the stance of the individual art therapist. As discussed in Chapter 1 in connection with the identity of the art therapist, the art therapist may lean heavily on both theory and prac-tice developed by the more established professions. In my view, it is incumbent upon the profession of art therapy to tap the creativity inherent in the work of its individual practitioners to develop new understandings and new forms. I will discuss this idea further under the systems that follow.

NATIONAL SERVICE SYSTEM

The discussion of the politics of art therapy at the facility and professional organization level has been somewhat downbeat. In fact on occasion I have told inquirers that I have found art therapy a wonderful way to work but a difficult profession. It is with the larger picture in mind, however, that I believe art therapy can become a wonderful profession as well. Art therapists are creative people, and organized art therapy has demon-strated enormous energy and accomplishment. When these characteris-tics are brought to bear on the larger frameworks in which all the rest reside, we will see the impact at every level.

The national service system structures treatment. Certain kinds of fa-cilities are provided. Those treated are designated by specific classifica-tions. Treatment adheres to certain forms and times. This system is not a static one. We have seen the changes brought about by tranquilizing medications, the community mental health movement, and the development of milieu therapy, to name only a few changes of the past several decades. It is possible for art therapists to contribute innovative input to this evolving system. There may be new forms of treatment, new centers for working with people (other than the usual hospitals, schools, clinics), new time frames, new kinds of spaces. To cite an obvious example, the 50 minute hour in an office may not be the best time and place for art therapy, and in fact many art therapists structure their work differently. Yet art therapy needn't adhere to the art studio model either. There may be ways of working yet to be developed that art therapists will create for the most efficacious manner to conduct art therapy as both a contribution to the service delivery system and as a further definition of art therapy by art therapists rather than by others.

PREVAILING SOCIAL ATTITUDES

Social attitudes determine definitions of mental illness, emotional disturbance, positive growth, and notions of how these conditions should be handled. This prevailing sea of ideas in which all our systems float is one of variety and flux. For example, at present we exist among both a medical model and a holistic health model. Any particular case may be understood and treated differently by practitioners of these two approaches.

Here again art therapists may have a contribution to make. We view our clients from a slightly different vantage point from others. We see and try to understand their imagery. We tap into a different sort of inner experience, processing of information, and communication compared with the usual verbal mode. From the art therapists' unique perspective may come significant understandings of human functioning and new approaches in aiding human growth.

These social and political forces are the background of our work. All too often we are so caught up in our everyday struggles and gratifications that we pay them little attention. But if art therapy is to reach its full potential, we who must work toward that goal need to expand our vision to regard art therapy in its fullest context.

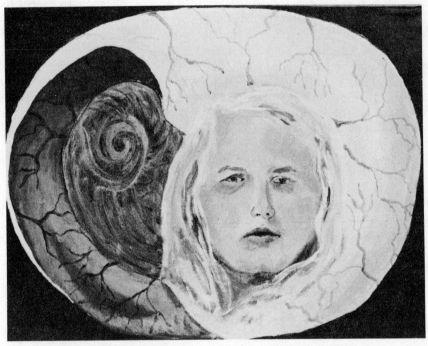

Figure 151. Pursuit of the Image: Self portrait with shell and roots or veins.

CHAPTER 12

Art as Therapy and Art Psychotherapy

Historically there has been a split within the art therapy profession. At times it has seemed more pronounced than others. The split began in a division of approach by its founding mothers, Margaret Naumburg and Edith Kramer, as evidenced in their writings (specifically Naumburg, 1966; and Kramer, 1971). This division was given formal recognition in the First Great Debate at the American Art Therapy Association's Annual Conference in 1982 (see Wadeson, 1982a).

I am devoting a separate chapter to this issue because it is one about which there has been much misunderstanding, often brought about by an unnatural polarization and unfounded generalizations. I have placed it in the section on Context of Art Therapy because both philosophical foundations of this argument and their more conspicuous political ramifications are part of art therapists' heritage.

Briefly stated, Kramer emphasizes the healing properties of art-making, its potentiality for aiding integration and synthesis, its role in sublimation, and the resulting lack of necessity for verbal interpretation or insight. Kramer is concerned with artistic quality (1975). Naumburg considers art symbolic language and is more interested in unraveling its meaning, depending more on verbal interpretation, insight, and transference, with less focus on artistic quality. Both pioneers operate within a psychoanalytic framework. A very important aspect of the comparison of these two pioneers' work is often lost from sight. Some art therapists, neglecting the context of Kramer's work, fail to recognize that she has worked primarily with children, despite the titles of her major works, both of which make the population explicit (*Art as Therapy with Children,* 1971, and *Childhood Art Therapy,* 1979).

Nevertheless, there are art therapists who generalize the principles of her work to all populations under all circumstances. It is obvious that one would work with children differently than with adults, and development of insight would be handled differently with young children.

Some art therapists describe themselves as using "art as therapy" and others describe themselves as "art psychotherapists." These terms used ontext of what I consider to be an artificial polarity are misleading. Having written a book entitled *Art Psychotherapy,* I am considered to be an "art psychotherapist," and yet there are frequent occasions when I use "art as therapy." Art certainly is therapy for me in my own work on myself. I have seen patients who never develop much insight through their art, yet certainly benefitted from the work. I did not choose the title *Art Psychotherapy* to distinguish it from "art as therapy." As stated in the *preface* to that book, art psychotherapists are those art therapists who are prepared to accept primary therapeutic responsibility rather than to work in an adjunctive capacity only. Either primary or adjunctive art therapy might be "art as therapy" or insight-oriented, or both.

I believe the art therapist must be guided by clients' needs and whatever conditions her place of work imposes. "Art as therapy" would be the more appropriate approach for those incapable of insight as well as those who develop sufficient emotional connection to art-making to benefit from the release of feeling and synthesizing potential of this process. I have worked with many clients who have made full use of both aspects of the work. There were those who were more amenable to "art as therapy" during certain periods and to an insight-oriented approach at another.

On the other hand, I have worked with others who had no interest in art nor were they in treatment long enough to develop themselves in art expression. Nevertheless, they gained much insight from relatively minimal drawings that exhibited no artistic quality in Kramer's terms. As one previously cited patient remarked, "At first I thought art therapy was silly and childish, but I really got a lot out of making these pictures even though I never did learn to draw." Some art therapists, gratified by their own art expression and exploration, presume that all clients eventually can and will want to do likewise. Immersing oneself in art-making is not everyone's metier, and art therapists should be sensitive to the routes that are the most liberating to any particular individual. That route might not necessarily be art, although for many, like the patient quoted here, release and insight may come from imagistic expression with an understanding art therapist.

EXAMPLE OF UNIFICATION OF APPROACH

Janet was a young woman I saw in private art therapy sessions who was able to make use of both "art as therapy" as well as insight-oriented art therapy. Figures 152 and 153 are examples of art expressions that facilitated insight. Both depend heavily on imagistic expressions with insight

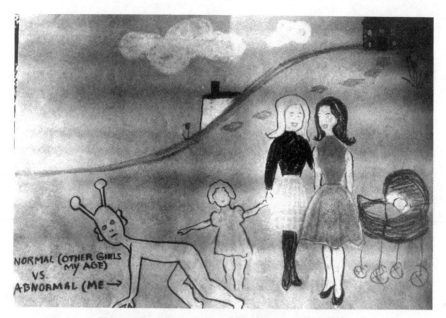

Figure 152. Janet's experience of herself growing up.

and self-exploration amplified by visual metaphors. In Figure 152 we see Janet's experience of herself growing up. Figure 153 is her father depicted as a clown with whom she identified. She said that he "performs" and is "obnoxious in front of others." She related his "repulsive" physical appearance to the scar on her belly from slashing herself when she "felt depressed when I wasn't seeing you." She saw the eyes as "hollow and death-like" and said she wanted to die and would take sleeping pills to get attention. She related the nose to the plastic surgery she had had on her nose some years previously. She also saw herself as the seal and said she had picked up some of her father's ways of performing and that they both get depressed, unlike her mother. The title, she said, is a song about a performer doing cartwheels and a spinning world. The grim-looking clown appears incongruously gaily dressed and as though he may have difficulty going through the hoop. In many ways this was an accurate representation of Janet and facilitated her recognition of her identification with her father, as well as her feelings toward him.

The title "King" for Figure 154 designates the tall bird Janet drew first before deciding to add his "family." She drew the bird on the left last and

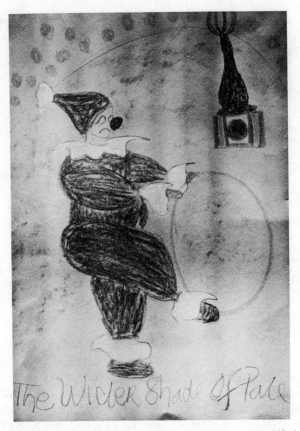

Figure 153. Janet's father as a clown with whom she identified.

said it was the prettiest. She called it "Little Fluff" and spoke of it affectionately as being the only one that was the same color as the father, whom she identified with her psychiatrist. The mother bird represents me and the other little birds are our other patients. She maintained over and over again, "He does care about Little Fluff," whom she described as tagging along and acting sort of dizzy. She became very attached to "Little Fluff," displaying an affection for the loveable child in herself for the first time (in contrast with Figure 152). "King" probably combines "story-telling or fantasy as therapy" with "art as therapy." Her attempt to create a family in therapy is apparent as is the contrast between "King" and the clown.

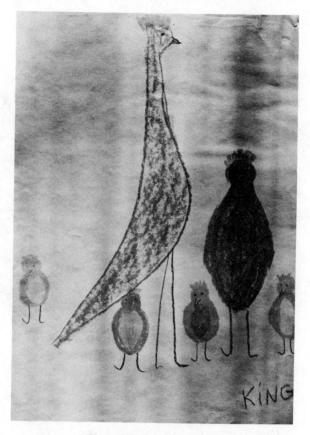

Figure 154. Janet in therapy.

Like Figure 154, "Menagerie," Figure 155, has a loveable-animal theme. The colors are more intense, and we can see a more imaginative use of space. Janet had no particular insights about this picture. It is much more clearly "art as therapy." She captured the whimsey of Figure 154, but this drawing depicts a bold and original style. She appeared to derive much satisfaction from it. Many of her earlier pictures had been full of anguish, depression, and self-loathing. The gaiety of "Menagerie" probably would not have been possible had she not progressed in dealing with the earlier, incapacitating view she had of herself.

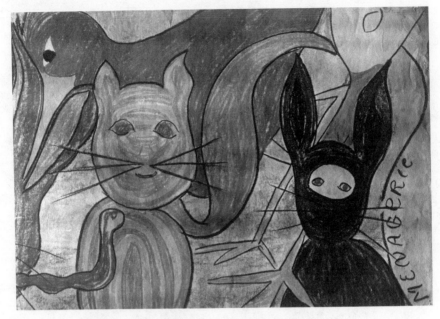

Figure 155. Janet using art as therapy.

ART AS THERAPY WITH A CHILD

Although I enjoy working with patients in an insight-oriented way, I have certainly worked with those for whom insight played a small or nonexistent part. (Mr. Gump, discussed in Chapter 3, is an example.) Like Edith Kramer's work with children, my work with that population has more often been art and relationship as therapy rather than insight-oriented art therapy. Mark is an example. At six-years-old he was diagnosed minimally brain-damaged after his mother and teacher reported disruptive behavior. Having my full attention in individual art therapy sessions, he was never disruptive and felt free to express some of the conflicts that disturbed him. In Figure 14 (Chapter 2), he displays both his identification with and fear of aggression. He told the following story about the picture: The whale has been shot with flaming arrows by a nice fisherman. He then amended the story, saying he had shot the whale and that it would be stuffed for a museum. The whale looked angry, he said. Mark changed the story again saying that he was just pretending that he shot the whale. In fantasizing about his aggressive image, he was trying to deal with his ambivalence. Interestingly, until becoming focused in creating his angry-looking whale, Mark had been depressed and self-punitive in the session, making several unsuccessful attempts to complete a picture, Figure 67. His self-deprecation ceased, however, when he allowed himself to express himself more aggressively through his whale. In talking about it, however, he still needed to undo, as he had in previous attempts to draw.

PURSUIT OF THE IMAGE

"Art psychotherapy," or what I prefer to designate the "insight-oriented" approach, is discussed at some length in Chapter 5, so in this chapter I would like to pursue "art as therapy" a bit further.

Art therapists risk losing some of art therapy's most valuable treasures at either end of the extremes of overreliance and underreliance on the verbal amplification of the art. I have written elsewhere (in this volume and in other works) about the underreliance on the art-maker's commentary. In such circumstances erroneous interpretations are frequently made, often secured by the interpreter's frame of reference. Much of this sort of "mind reading" could be avoided by a sensitive questioning of the art's author (See Chapter 5).

On the other hand, there is sometimes an overreliance on verbalization. I believe this sort of short shrift of the image disturbs those who practice "art as therapy." It certainly concerns me when I see students miss what I find to be art therapy's unique power by relegating the image to the place of a mere stepping stone to a verbal exchange. As result, I have recently developed a workshop to aid art therapists in exploring the image's potential.

The workshop is titled, "Pursuit of the Image." After a period of meditation in which the mind is allowed to wander, participants develop an image in whatever medium they choose. In small groups, usually of four, they explore their art expressions. Instead of giving each other the usual explanations, they refrain from explaining and instead search for what they find exciting, surprising, puzzling, or intriguing in their own work. The others then respond to one's art expression in the same way, rather than to try to understand it. The small groups then separate and each person creates another art expression drawn from what was found intriguing in the first one. This may be prompted by one's own reaction or stimulated by reactions from the group. The small groups form again and a similar discussion ensues. The process is repeated again with a third art expression drawn from the second. The workshop is completed with a review of all the art and the entire process in the small groups.* Usually these art expressions and discussions take about half a day, but the process can be continued indefinitely, and it may also be carried out alone with self-reflection instead of discussion.

There are two features of this format that depart from the usual art therapy procedures. Most significant is developing the image through a succession of renditions, each inspired by its predecessor. The second departure alters the verbal processing to minimize the intellectual and enhance emotional response.

The following is an example of the process in my own "pursuit of the image" begun alone, continued in a group, and completed alone. In this case it was also combined with another expressive art form, poetry-writing. I have chosen this example because it is closely related to the writing of this book. Just before leaving the University of Illinois at Chicago to return to my home in Washington, D.C. for a winter quarter sabbatical leave to write this book, I wrote a poem in anticipation. It was a winter turning inwards and a going home.

HIBERNATION

The inward curve
of the spiraled shell
is cupped to contain a whisper
the way my hand holds my breath
to your ear.
The secret is winter
wrapped in soft blankets
its sounds hushed
in weightless down.
The whisper is a lullabye
singing me to sleep
deep within the earth.
The spiraled shell is myself
curving inward, outward,
in undulating rhythms
of surging tides.
This is the season to go home
far within myself,

* I am indebted to Abby Calisch for the idea of successive drawings based on one another demonstrated at the Third Annual University of Illinois Art Therapy Conference, 1984, in her "Problem Solving Through Art Therapy" workshop.

to turn away from bird cries
echoing in my ear.
Outer garments fall to my feet
in dried husks
as I wrap myself in winter silence
and curl into its rooty hollows.
Winter wear is a dress of dreams
dotted with snowdrops
that blossom in strange profusion
beneath the silent drifting snows.
The journey home is solitary, soft, and still.
Slowly I spiral in.

That poem was in my mind when I meditated in a Pursuit of the Image workshop. Figure 156 arose from my image of hibernating beneath the snow. Most intriguing to me were the roots that became more prominent in the painting than in the poem where they are mentioned only once as "rooty hollows." So in the second picture I painted the roots, Figure 157. They looked to me as though they were reaching down for something but I did not know what. The book title, *The Heart of Darkness,* came to my mind, but I didn't mention it to my group. One of its members turned my painting upside-down and said that what intrigued her about it was that it looked like arteries and veins. Her association coincided with mine and I pursued it in my final picture, Figure 158, in which the roots reach for a

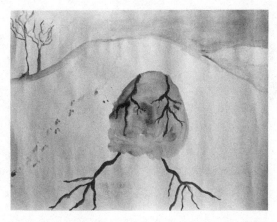

Figure 156. Pursuit of the Image: Hibernating under the snow.

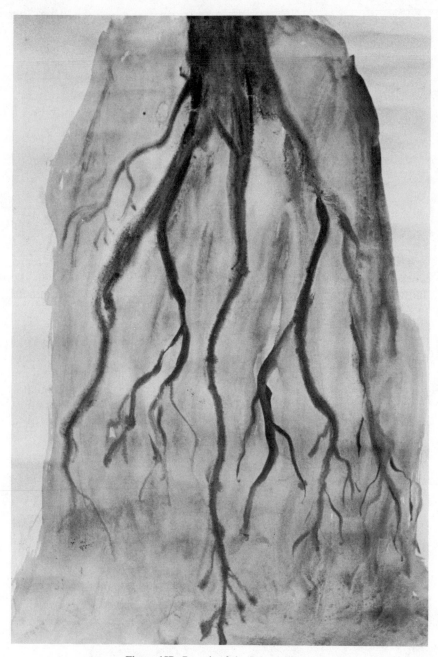

Figure 157. Pursuit of the Image: Roots.

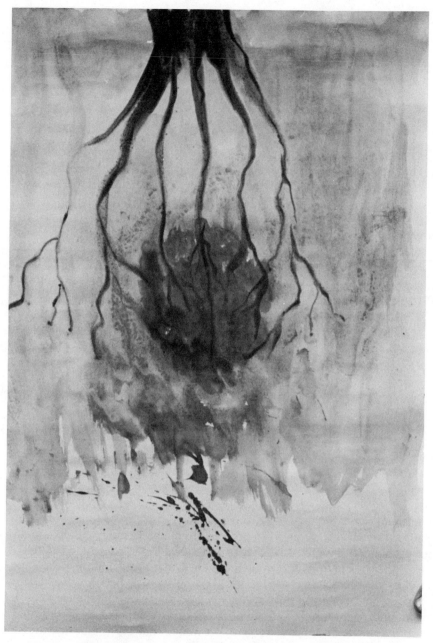

Figure 158. Pursuit of the Image: Reaching for the heart.

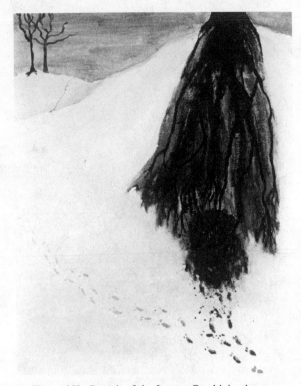

Figure 159. Pursuit of the Image: Combining images.

heart and red blood courses through them. After the workshop the water painted images still did not feel finished to me so I combined them in an acrylic painting, Figure 159. Finally I returned to the poem and painted a self-portrait superimposed on a spiral shell that at the end became covered by root-like veins (see Figure 151).

My process evolved through unexpected images, spontaneous in both poem and paintings. They had much to say to me about where I found myself at that time, particularly the meaning that the roots, heart, and blood held for me. It was not through interpretations or explanations that my art spoke to me, but through the imagery. I ended feeling more deeply in touch with myself.

CONCLUSION

In this chapter, I have emphasized the "art as therapy" aspect of my work because I have become identified as an "art psychotherapist" with the inaccurate connotation that I use the art only for assessment or insight. In my other writings, as well as in sections of this book, there is a greater focus on insight and revelation of the inner experience (Chapters 4, 5, 6). I hope that the examples presented here make apparent that I believe the art therapist must be responsive and sensitive to the client's needs and proclivities and flexible in her encouragement of directions for work. She is neither art teacher nor verbal therapist, but is uniquely an art therapist. As such, she utilizes both "art as therapy" and "art psychotherapy," rather than only one or the other.

The question has been posed to art therapists: "Are you an artist or a therapist?" (Ault, 1977). The artificial polarity of "art as therapy" and "art psychotherapy" is not only embodied in this question, but is seen in the split in the term "art therapy" itself, with some art therapists seeming more at home with the "art" and others with the "therapy." Perhaps the amalgamation of art and therapy is still too recent for its seam not to show. As training continues to develop and improve, art therapists will feel equally at home in both worlds and particularly in the unique and newer world of art therapy. The next chapter looks to the training that is grounded in both art and therapy but is uniquely art therapy. As identity of "art therapist" becomes strengthened, the either or-*ness* of "artist" or "therapist" and "art as therapy" and "art psychotherapy" will become a nonissue.

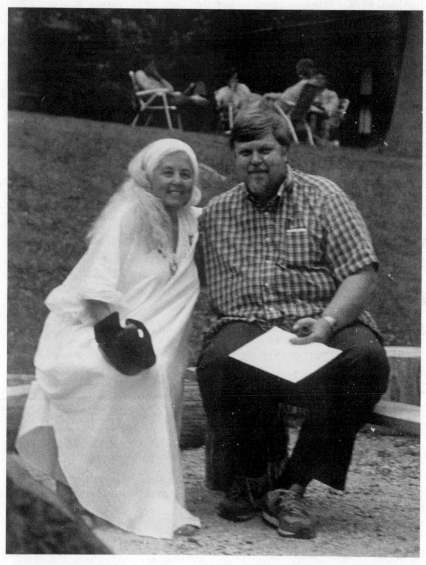

Figure 160. The author with well-known art therapist and educator Robert Ault.

CHAPTER 13

Art Therapy Training

Training to be an art therapist is a life-long process in which the art therapist utilizes her experience to heighten her sensitivity and seeks opportunity for new learning both in formal settings, such as attending conferences and workshops, and informally through stretching her own approaches to her work. The basics, however, are usually gained through established training programs to prepare the professional art therapist. The field is still sufficiently young to be populated also by some "old timers," such as myself, who entered art therapy before the first training programs were developed around 1970. Although the usual route to professional art therapy is through a master's degree in art therapy or in art, education, or psychology with a concentration in art therapy, there are also other avenues one might take, such as a clinically based training program (in contrast to university based training).

Presently the only credentialing in the field is registration by the American Art Therapy Association which awards the letters ATR to signify "art therapist registered." The simplest route to registration is a master's degree from a program "approved" by the American Art Therapy Association plus 1000 hours of paid art therapy experience. The AATA approves programs that demonstrate through a lengthy self-evaluation process that they meet the Association's guidelines for education and training. Registration may also be granted through other combinations of education and experience.

Rather than detailing the various training possibilities, I will give only a brief outline of basics and then concentrate on the art therapy training process and the results I believe it should achieve.

BASICS OF TRAINING

As stated throughout this book, the art therapist is first and foremost a therapist. Therefore, she needs all the preparation any professional psychotherapist trained at the master's degree level requires. This clinical

273

foundation includes courses in human growth and development through-out the entire life cycle, psychopathology, clinical methods, and an intro-duction to various theoretical bases for clinical approaches (such as psy-choanalysis, Jungian analytical psychology, gestalt therapy, and so forth). Because art therapists are often called upon to conduct group and family therapy, courses in group dynamics and family dynamics are also neces-sary.

Some art therapy graduate training programs do not require these ba-sics but relegate some or all of this subject matter to prerequisites. In my experience, art therapy program applicants have often retained little knowledge from their prerequisites. As part of their art therapy training, on the other hand, their objectives are more purposeful and they are able to integrate theory with application. Graduate level professional educa-tion is certainly able to take advantage of the opportunity of relating theory to practice in ways that general undergraduate courses may not be able to do. For a practicing professional, theoretical knowledge is of little use if it does not inform practice.

Naturally, all art therapy education provides training specific to art therapy. This should include history, general principles (there is not art therapy theory), methods, and specializations. A background such as this may be organized into courses in various ways, and different training programs have different emphases. Nevertheless, upon completion of training, a student should understand the development of the profession and its relation to the fields of psychology, psychiatry, education, art; how to plan and conduct art therapy with various populations, individu-ally, in groups and families; and how to approach and understand art made in art therapy, including a background in developmental stages in art expression. In a two year full-time training program (the length of time necessary for most art therapy master's degrees) it is not feasible to cover every possible population in depth, so there should be an emphasis on basic principles and an opportunity for students to specialize through electives in areas of their interests. Nevertheless, among the basics should be included work with groups, families, children, and emotionally disturbed adults. A survey conducted by the American Art Therapy Asso-ciation's Research Committee indicated that 75 percent of all art thera-pists work with the latter population.

Carefully supervised practicum work is the oven in which the training bread is baked. Most students find their hands-on work with clients and patients the most meaningful and gratifying part of their training. The AATA requires 600 hours of supervised field work, but because of its importance the program I direct requires more. I believe also that students should be placed in at least two different kinds of settings (for example, a hospital and a school) with two different kinds of populations (such as outpatients in an urban clinic and the elderly in a residential home) in order to give them perspective. I believe also that at least one placement should offer opportunity for long-term work so that the student can learn what it's like to be almost a part of a facility's staff and to have the possibility of following clients over time.

The arrangement of supervision varies from program to program. I have found a combination of both faculty and field supervision with both small group and individual sessions to be most comprehensive. In some training programs, students secure their own field placements, and as a result the field supervisor may have had no prior association with the training program. Since supervision is such a crucial dimension of the training, I believe supervisors must be selected carefully. The arrangement I have developed entails a careful screening of placement sites with much information exchanged regarding our program and expectations of the facility. Often our field supervisors are not art therapists, but other mental health professionals, such as psychiatrists, psychologists, or social workers (at the master's level or above). The student meets with the field supervisor for at least one regularly scheduled hour-long individual session weekly and with a faculty art therapist supervisor for a two-hour small group meeting in which there is opportunity for learning and sharing from other students. The faculty supervisor visits the placement and communicates with the field supervisor as needed and provides the student with individual supervision biweekly as well.

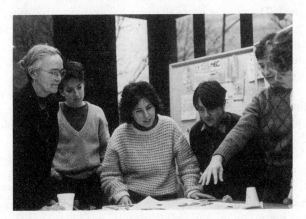

Figure 161. An art therapy supervision group, led by Evadne McNeil (left), discusses the patients' art from sessions the students conduct.

Most master's degree programs require a thesis. Sometimes it is a research project. I have found research in a two-year training program to be an unrealistic goal. Two years is hardly enough time to prepare a clinician, much less a competent researcher as well. Much of the student-conducted research projects I have read (in submission for AATA's annual research award) have been insubstantial and often poorly conceived. Nevertheless, they have been encouraged, I believe, because art therapists hope that research will lend credibility to the profession. (I will discuss the plan for research in training at the end of this chapter.) My students are required to compete a final project "comparable to a thesis," but not of a research design. Often they tackle an issue for independent study that has grown out of their practicum experience. The purpose is to help to develop their critical thinking, their ability to integrate concepts and experience, their focusing, and their capacity to develop a solution to a problem they have posed. Writing and presenting the material is also excellent preparation for such professional activities. A number of art therapy graduates have published and presented their projects at professional conferences.

PROCESS OF TRAINING

The organization of training previously described forms its skeleton. The heart of training is self-awareness. This is why preparation to become an art therapist is so demanding. The student must not only undertake a full academic schedule but also a journey into the self, often a far more difficult ordeal. The results more than compensate for the effort. I call this the heart of the work not only for its centrality but also because of the strong feelings aroused.

It is important that much art therapy training be experiential. Intellectual apperception gained by observing from without through reading or listening to a lecturer is distant and less involving than an individual's being centered in an experience which can directly pull on one's feelings. Experiential learning can be operationalized by students role playing both patients and art therapists as one aspect of enhancing self awareness. Whether the role is a false one (such as playing a psychotic adolescent or alcoholic indigent) or not, one cannot help but be oneself, even in the role. Both "patients" and "therapists" learn a great deal in the process. Recently in a class I portrayed a paranoid psychotic. I was amazed at how readily I was bound by my own idiosyncratic world and how little the "art therapist's" interventions meant to me unless they clicked into my own

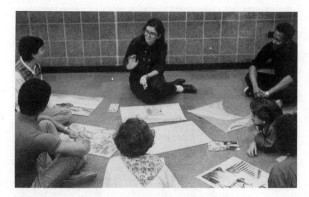

Figure 162. In order to experience the group art therapy process, students form a small group and share the feelings expressed in their drawings.

unique experience. It was another confirmation of the importance of the therapist's sensitivity to the client's state, and of course the one who plays therapist gains a great deal from the feedback from both her "patient" and the other students and teacher who observe. Such exercises enhance both personal and professional self-awareness.

In the group art therapy class I teach, students use the class group as the model for applying their understanding of group dynamics. Painfully for some, they come to see their own interaction in a group. For many, this is the most emotionally stressful course they take as they deal with issues of competition, relationship to authority, and group factions.

In a final class I teach on termination, students not only deal with their termination from clients they are seeing in their field placements, but also they must reflect on and plan their own termination from the training program and their transition from student to professional. Much of this work entails a review of their entire training. They reread the journal they have kept throughout, present to the class their growth through the art they have made, and reflect on their initial reasons for wanting to become art therapists (written at the outset of the program). They also use class time to fill in any gaps in training they may perceive. Students take leadership in this enterprise to prepare them to be responsible for their own education following graduation.

In the course of much art therapy class work, students make art to try out art therapy exercises. This is necessary to grasp what it is like to be a participant in art therapy, thereby enhancing their empathy and understanding of their clients. Thus, they may try the "scribble technique," a

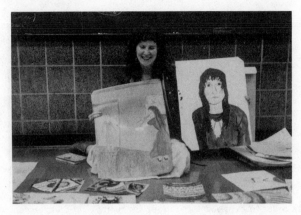

Figure 163. Art therapy student Lynn Lidbury reviews the art she has made as part of her training to examine her own personal and professional development.

drawing of a dream, a picture of their family of origin, a representation of the group, a group mural, a mask, a clay form of their present feelings, and so forth. They are then called upon to "process" their art expressions to whatever extent they feel comfortable. From the making of the art, reflecting upon it, sharing it with classmates, and hearing comments from the others in the class, self-awareness advances.

Related to personal self-awareness is professional self-awareness. In this context I mean understanding the world view one brings to the work. Some training programs offer a particular orientation (psychoanalytic, for example). I believe students should be familiar with the major theoretical orientations and therapeutic approaches. As conducting therapy is such a personal endeavor, one must select knowledge and methods that are consonant with one's own belief system and values. This is a dynamic process that continues throughout one's entire professional life. It is a reciprocal venture, because the training, the acquisition of new knowledge and experience, may influence one's belief system and values as well. Thus for students in the program I direct, a major task is the integration of many sources of knowledge and experience.

Understanding of self is expanded to understanding of clients and patients. One does not truly understand in a personal and human way through abstractions or generalities. By recalling feelings of estrangement I begin to grasp my patient's sense of isolation. By remembered feelings of helplessness and the resultant anger I experienced, I begin to see my patient's rage at an enforced hospitalization. It is in this way that students are encouraged to know those with whom they work. Self comes first.

Because the developing self-awareness that has been described is a shared experience, art therapy training tends to be very intense and intimate. My hope is that each class will become a learning community whose members offer one another not only the stimulation of their shared experience and the diversity each contributes, but also support for the self-with-others process that therapy is all about. It is very clear to me that learning comes from many sources—not only books and teachers, but clients and students as well. It is also clear that learning prospers where there is both challenge and support. Learning requires stretching, exposure to the unfamiliar, efforts at mastery. These can be precarious experiences. Risking the swing from the flying trapeze is easier with a net below. Students come to realize that there is much they can receive from one another. In many instances they begin to develop colleagues during their training who will continue to offer professional support for years to come.

Beyond developing relationships with other art therapy students, those in the program I direct are also encouraged in their relationships with the other mental health professionals with whom they work at practicum sites. Art therapy is a young profession, so the art therapy student may provide a facility's first exposure to the profession. In fact, art therapy training programs have been in the vanguard of the expansion of the field, offering free art therapy services in the form of its student placements.

Many facilities where a treatment program was begun in this manner have subsequently hired an art therapist in order to make art therapy a permanent part of their services. It has been through student placements as well that the field has expanded into new areas. For example, the program I direct has developed practicum training beyond the usual psychiatric and school settings to include the city jail, child-life programs, physical rehabilitation, facilities for the elderly, half-way houses, community centers, child abuse programs, and so forth. Offering the first master's degree training in both Houston and Chicago, the programs I directed were frequently contacted by facilities requesting a student. When first starting, however, both programs had to make the effort to attract facilities for practicum placements. In both cases, it has been incumbent upon the students to educate the staffs about art therapy and in a sense become ambassadors for the profession. Given art therapy's still youthful position among the mental health services, this sort of art therapy ombudsmanship is an important part of a student's experience. Students must learn to describe art therapy and demonstrate it to other professionals. They must learn to be able to present their work at staff meetings and to provide in-service presentations or workshops for staff. They must learn appropriate ways to involve other staff in their work so that co-workers will be facilitating of their efforts in particular and come to value art therapy in general. I frequently tell students that working with patients is easy. It's working with the staff that's difficult. Therefore, a significant aspect of training in the field is learning to operate within an institution. Institutional practices sometimes come as a shock, so there is often much soul-searching (more self-awareness) that constitutes this aspect of the work as well.

CREATIVITY AND ART

If self-awareness is the heart of learning art therapy, then creativity and art are its connective tissue. The two are interconnected as creativity enhances self-awareness through personal art projects and self-awareness enhances creativity through expressing deeper layers of the self. Specifically, in order to promote creativity in the training program I direct, students are required to produce creative art projects in lieu of taking exams and writing papers (although these learning and evaluation procedures are used in some instances as well). The creative projects serve the purpose of promoting cognition and integration as well.* The same principles that operate in art therapy are applied to art therapy training: The student learns to use the materials of visual expression to solve problems in learning in the same way the client solves them in therapy. As the basis of art therapy is the translation of experience into art expression, it is a practice I wish to stimulate and encourage.

We can expect that those training to become art therapists are visually-oriented people who are accustomed to integrating experience through art expression. In that they come to us particularly articulate in this area, they usually welcome and enjoy the opportunity to draw together their learning through the art-making process. Just as is the case with clients and patients, the narcissistic cathexis to creative work enables the student to become involved in learning on a deeper level, and the sense of achievement enhances the confidence needed by the beginning art therapist. Further, the teacher is aided in gaining a clear view of the student's learning because, as in client artwork, discrepancies or areas of difficulty show up readily in the visual product. In addition, the art therapy teacher is challenged with unique and original solutions to assignments. The joy and enthusiasm she derives from her students' creativity is a far cry from

---

* Pat Allen and I presented some of this material at the American Art Therapy Association Annual Conference, 1982. See Allen and Wadeson, (1982).

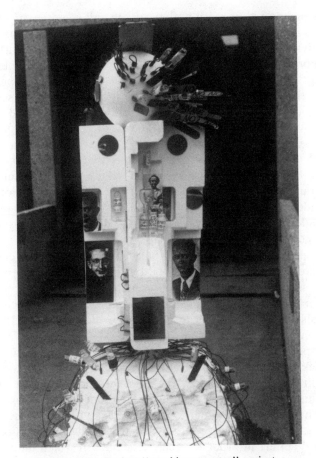

Figure 164. Student "psychic apparatus" project.

what is often the tedium of reading papers and grading tests. In this way (as well as in other aspects of teaching) I feel enlivened by my work and bring a vitality of approach to the teaching/learning experience.

An example of the way in which an art project facilitates cognition is exemplified in Figure 164 representing a model of Freud's psychic apparatus of id, ego, and superego.* To create such a representation, a deeper understanding is required than might be necessary in writing a paper or taking an exam in which one could parrot the lingo of a text on the

* This assignment was developed by Pat Allen in a course on History and Theory of Art Therapy.

subject. Constructed primarily of styrofoam and standing approximately three feet high, the three components of the psychic apparatus in Figure 164 are divided as follows: id—base, a multilayered irregularly shaped form to represent chaos with wires to suggest sensation and feelings, vials containing "libidinal juices," a knife for the castration complex, and a screw for the oedipal complex; ego—the head with compass eyes for searching out directions, tongue depressors labeled "yes" and "no" that can be moved out of the ego and stabbed into the id and repressed, a paddle to represent defense mechanisms, and a teeter-totter holding marbles for the reaction formation defense mechanism; super-ego—central column with photos of parents (introjects), books for injunctions learned in the library of memory, and mirrors representing introjection, projection, and identification. The possibility of moving objects from one area to another indicated the student's grasp of the dynamic relationship among the three constructs of the psychic apparatus.

It is evident from this example that many aspects of psychoanalytic theory were operationally understood by this student. I believe that not only does such a project reflect the student's learning, the process of its production fosters a comprehension of concepts and experience. Such art projects also enable students to personalize their learning. In studying Jungian concepts, students made masks of their own "shadow" and "personna" aspects (Figure 165). This project encourages personal self-exploration, making conceptual integration personally meaningful.

Rudolph Arnheim considers the arts the most valuable means of strengthening perception, without which productive thinking is impossible (Arnheim, 1969). In order to make an idea visible its essential traits must be grasped. Abraham Maslow proposes that all education be conducted through art in order to create a society in which individuals are able to improvise (Maslow, 1977). Thus these two leading thinkers of our time would expand the use of art for learning beyond education in art and art therapy.

In addition to cognition of concepts, students must learn to grasp process. For the final project from the group art therapy course I teach, students represent the dynamic process of their class group's evolution and their own part in it. This is an interesting assignment in that students must show development over time. It teaches them to be aware of process. Further, this multidimensional assignment necessitates a concomitant self-awareness in relation to the larger group process. The perspectives required for this project are those needed by the group therapist.

In an innovative approach to this problem, Marcy Baranchik used the metaphor of record albums to express group themes and colored the

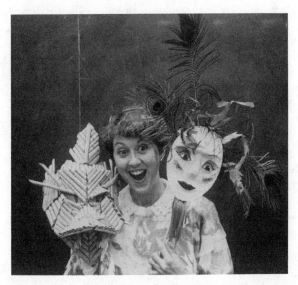

Figure 165. Claudia Clennard with her "shadow" and "personna" masks.

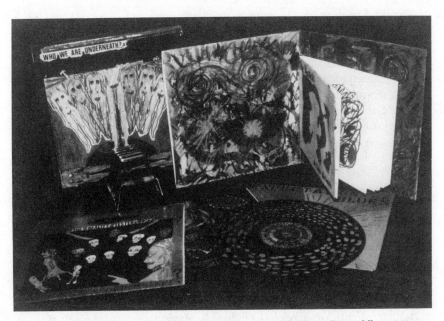

Figure 166. Student group art therapy project by Marcy Baranchik.

inside, the record, to reveal her own process, Figure 166. Each record represented a different group session with the group's theme for the meeting given an often humorous title and picture. Such subjects as sexuality, relationship to authority, peer relations, and so forth, were the content. Music was an apt metaphor. Especially interesting was the inside-outside relationship of record to album cover to show her own inner relationship to the external process. Some of the drawings on the records were quite personal. The series of albums showed the group's development and progression.

Beyond cognition and process comprehension is the necessity for an even broader integration of learning. Integration requires a sorting and relating of one thing to another. Art therapy students are bombarded with a tremendous amount of new learning. It is essential that they understand theory, make it meaningful to themselves, operationalize it into practice and from practice evolve new theoretical understandings in an ever-spiraling loop. A synthesis of all this learning requires reflection out of which new relationships are juxataposed and new awarenesses emerge. For the artistically inclined individual, the art-making process is a natural vehicle for such synthesizing. The economy of art, the message of metaphor, can condense in a personal, expressive image, the integration that has occurred.

The final project for an art therapy clinical methods course I teach is a representation of what the student has learned. This is an interesting assignment in that one cannot possibly convey all that has been learned. A selection is required. And a reflection is required—a determination of what has been most significant. That which is selected must be expressed in a form that holds together and communicates. Projects such as this illustrate that not everyone learns the same thing nor in the same way. This acknowledgment is at the foundation of all art therapy effort and efficacy. Art therapy's value of the uniqueness of individual expression is integral to its special impact.

Use of Art-Making in Supervision

Art-making to enhance the art therapy student's self-awareness and learning can aid supervision as well. The supervisee can illustrate clients, her relationship with them, problematic staff relationships (Figure 167), images of the facility in which she works, feelings about her work, career goals, and so forth. Art can also be used for feedback from supervision group members. In a supervision group, members can role-play work with particular clients or invented clients displaying particular problems. A

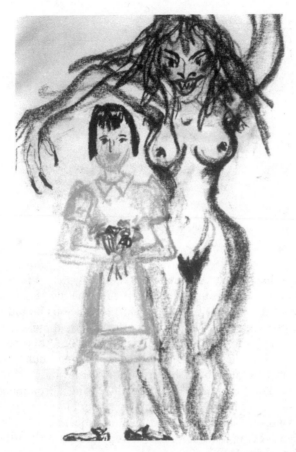

Figure 167. A split view of a staff member with whom an art therapist was having a problematic relationship.

group member can actually conduct a brief art therapy session with another member. After the session, "therapist," "patient," and group observers each make a picture of the interaction. In this way, the usual verbal comments are augmented by imagery and metaphor that may tap unconscious reactions. Sometimes there is a powerful concordance of imagery despite lack of discussion prior to the quick and spontaneous art-making responses. For example, in some instances all group members have used the same color to represent the client and the same different color to represent the therapist. Similar shapes have emerged as well. Dimensions of closeness and distance, representations of affect, power,

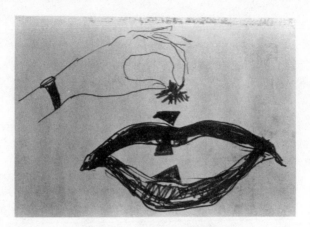

Figure 168. Art used for supervision.

control, strengths and weaknesses are readily displayed in a quick picture. Sometimes a surprising metaphor is illuminating. For example, an observer drew the "patient" in harem garb for reasons he did not understand. As he processed his picture, he realized he had picked up some of the seductive ways the "patient" was relating to the "therapist." Figure 168 is a quick drawing I made as observer of one such session. The "patient" is represented by a large mouth, somewhat down-turned in dissatisfaction. The "therapist" is the hand wearing a prominent watch as she keeps order and time. She is dropping little tidbits into the "patient," hardly a substantial meal. This sort of imagistic response is far more powerful in conveying a sense of the therapeutic (or not so therapeutic) process than words alone.

ADVANCED TRAINING

At present the master's degree and the ATR credential are the terminal points in art therapy training and credentialing respectively. Nevertheless, many art therapists have sought Ph.D. degrees in related fields or an additional master's degree such as the masters in social work. The motivations have usually been enhanced practice opportunities, sometimes facilitated by third party payment, and academic positions. Many have pursued nontraditional or self-designed Ph.D. degrees in order to develop and further their art therapy learning. My background is not unusual in this regard. When my NIH position ended after many years, due to a general shift in its Adult Psychiatry Branch from psychodynamic investigations to biochemical studies, I realized that I would need additional credentialing to develop my private practice and to teach art therapy. I had been engaged in both with only a B.A. degree, but it was becoming increasingly obvious during the 1970s that credentialing standards were getting stricter. I sought the master's in social work degree in order to receive third-party payment (a suitable credential in Maryland where I was practicing) and a Ph.D. degree in order to teach in academia. I pursued a self-directed doctorate for the opportunity and encouragement it gave me to write the book I had been hoping to publish (Wadeson, 1980).

In 1979, a year after I received my doctorate degree, I became aware that more and more art therapists, particularly those in positions of leadership, were also seeking Ph.D. degrees, often in related fields. I was curious about the implications of this trend so I conducted an informal survey among the profession's leadership and presented the findings at AATA's 1979 Annual Conference (Wadeson, 1982). The results indicated that most sought doctorates for professional advancement and felt that the benefits were worth the effort. Most also considered an art therapy Ph.D. degree premature at that time.

Having as recently as this morning been consulted by an art therapist I supervise who is interested in further education to enhance her professional opportunities, I add the following soliloquy for the benefit of others who may be considering such a step:

WITH APOLOGIES TO UNCLE WILL

To Ph.D., or not to Ph.D.: that is the question:
Whether 'tis nobler in the mind to suffer
The slings and arrows of outrageous professional pressure
Or to shoot the finger to a sea of supervisors
And by opposing, offend them. To hesitate, to contemplate—
No more; and by forestalling to say we end
The credentialing pressures and the thousand clinical ambitions
The art therapist is heir to! 'Tis a consumation
Devoutly to be wished. To hesitate, to contemplate—
To contemplate—perchance to meditate; ay, there's the rub,
For in that meditation what fantasies may come
When we have shuffled off this professional ambition
Must give us pause; there's the respect
That makes calamity of so long career:
For who would bear the neglects of administrators,
The low pay, the proud doctor's contumely,

The pangs of despised charting, bureaucratic delay,
The insolence of office, and the spurns
From other professionals less worthy,
When she herself might her reputation make
With a bare sheepskin? But who would dull courses take,
To grunt and sweat under weary tomes,
To anguish in the dread of professors' scorn
And the inconclusive research, from whose frustrations
No doctoral candidate escapes unscathed, puzzles the will
And makes us rather bear the ills we have,
Than fly to others we know not of?
Thus wishy-washy ambivalence makes dilettantes of us all,
And thus the native hue of resolution
Is sicklied o'er with the pale cast of thought
And dissertations of great pitch and moment
With this regard of their currants turn awry
And loose the name of Doctorate

Art therapists are an ambitious lot. In the years since my survey, the trend toward additional advanced degrees has increased (despite the wisdom of the soliloquy). There seem to be two possible directions toward which this phenomenon can lead the art therapy profession. One is exemplified by an art therapist who is presently completing a degree from a school of professional psychology. Her specialty has been in work with children and her dissertation studies graphic indices of certain childhood experiences. In her clinical work prior to Ph.D. training, she gave the hospitalized children with whom she worked 8 ½" x 11" paper so that their pictures would fit into their charts. I believe this art therapist will become a child psychologist and that she will use art primarily as a testing instrument.

Another art therapist who has made significant contributions to the field both before and since her advanced training told me that when she opened her private practice recently, she announced herself as specializing in child therapy rather than in art therapy in order to attract more clientele.

On the other hand, there are many art therapists, particularly leaders in the field, who have remained identified as art therapists after obtaining advanced degrees in areas other than art therapy. My own direction has been determined by the excitement and creativity I find in art therapy and the challenge of being a part of the development of a young field.

The two possible directions I see fostered by increased advanced credentialing are the following: (1) A number of art therapists might move out of art therapy, using art as an adjunct to their work in clinical psychology or social work; (2) Or advanced training may lead to further development of art therapy, as I will discuss below. The possibility of the former is heightened by the greater opportunities and recognition accorded more established professions. Calling oneself "clinical psychologist" may bring more prestige than the title "art therapist" in addition to offering licensing and third-party payment possibilities. If art therapy becomes established as a "lower status" profession, it will attract fewer bright and creative people to its ranks, and those who begin in art therapy will be further motivated to move on to other professional disciplines.

The second direction is the more challenging one. Since many art therapists tend to seek advanced training, the movement I see would be toward the development of art therapy doctoral training. The 1979 survey indicated a general opinion that the field had not yet built up a sufficient body of knowledge to provide doctoral study. Yet it seems to me that Ph.D. candidates would be the very ones to develop the foundation work the profession so sorely needs.

Dissertations could be devoted to aspects of the theory-building which art therapists have heretofore neglected. Aesthetics, creativity, human development, and societal influences could be related to art therapy in ways to deepen our understanding of human functioning as revealed in art therapy. As mentioned previously, the art therapist's vantage point is a unique one, providing views of creative potential as well as experience processed imagistically. Utilizing the special information the art therapist gains in this way for the enlargement of understanding of human growth and pathology is a significant challenge in both theory building and research.

The research that many contend will add to the profession's credibility could be undertaken in a thorough-going way encompassing not only comprehensive training in behavioral science research methodology, but also encouragement toward the development of new methodological strategies to tap the unique data art expression provides. Established methodologies often reduce or neglect the richness of art expression, necessitating the creation of new systems for the collection and analysis of art therapy data.

Doctorate study might also serve to educate the educators. Experience in art therapy clinical work is a necessary condition for training art therapists, but certainly not a sufficient one. Clearly, education is an enterprise quite distinct from clinical work with its own special competencies.

Finally, a Ph.D. program might also provide advanced clinical work as well as training in administration and program development. In other words, all the areas that form the substantial base of doctorate study are most likely to be developed in the rigorous work demanded in writing a doctoral dissertation. Parallel to the way in which clinical work and psychological theory have developed hand in hand (Freud and Jung, for example), so art therapy theory and research development are more likely to accompany doctorate study programs than to precede them.

Were all these areas to be developed, art therapy would grow in substance, stature, and contribution to both the community and the general body of knowledge of human understanding. If past growth is a predictor, I believe this will happen. But we are still young and have a long way to go.

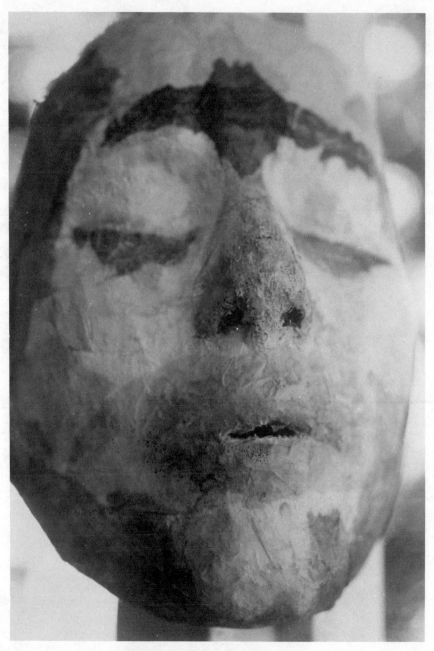

Figure 169. Mask made by the author.

CHAPTER 14

Beyond Art Therapy

A discussion of the Context of Art Therapy would not be complete without reference to concerns that transcend the boundaries of traditional art therapy. Therapy at its best is not simply the alleviation of symptoms and suffering. For many it provides the potential for wholeness, healing, and growth, the natural direction for a process that seeks the positive development of the whole person. Creation of an improved life leads inevitably to an expression of basic values and understandings of life itself. In this way, the therapeutic process borders the realms of the spiritual. In this light as well, the art therapy process evokes imagery to foster the individual's deeper connection with the universal.

This chapter is probably the book's most difficult to write. It deals with the ineffable. Art therapy process used for purposes "beyond therapy" border the netherlands transcending the boundaries of everyday existence into regions that might be variously named soul, spirituality, or meaning in life. For some of us, these are the realms of life's greatest poignancy, and they occupy large tracts of our existence. Others among us devote our energies elsewhere and may give little attention to existential questions. Most of us change over the course of our lives in both the kind and amount of interest we take in these matters.

The art therapy process is one of creating, understanding, and relating to imagery. In all these ways it offers potential for viewing the framework of our own existence. Realizations in the realms of "soul" or "spirit" seldom are delivered through rational processes. More often they involve emotional experiences, frequently accompanied by images, arriving unbidden. Religion, myths, philosophy, psychology all have attempted to answer questions surrounding our mortality. Visual metaphors have been a strong component of these often elaborate systems. Much of the world's great art has been created in the service of a relationship with the immortal. Think of the cathedrals of Europe, the pyramids of Egypt and Meso-America, the masks of the African Cameroons, the wood carvings of New Guinea, the totem poles of the Pacific Northwest.

You may object that I am speaking of art and not art therapy. "Art for

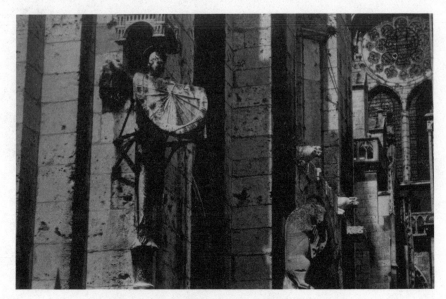

Figure 170. Angel sundial, Chartres cathedral, France.

art's sake" as we know it today is a relatively recent development for Western Civilization. At other times and in other places art was used for ritual, ceremony, tribute, and teaching. The illiterate serf who entered a church in Medieval Europe was humbled by its magnificence and reminded of important teachings as he followed the Station's of the Cross painted on its walls. An old Scandinavian church I visited recently has remnants of devil depictions in its underpainting, no doubt serving as a warning to the wayward and pious alike. American Indians and Australian Aboriginals created representations of family animal totems as reminders and tributes to the spirits that governed the family (Figure 171). The reclining statue of the Mayan Choc Moul received in his cupped hands the hearts cut from those sacrificed in tribute to him. (You may wonder what relation any of this has to the process of art therapy.)

Through imagistic forms people of various cultures throughout many ages have called upon art expressions both as representation and communication in their search for the meaning of their own existence. Prevailing ideologies created gods, spirits, sacred animals, holy places, and divine personages. More than any other form of expression, these creations were represented by visual art to inspire the culture's ideal of proper living and to bring it the benevolence of the powerful forces perceived to

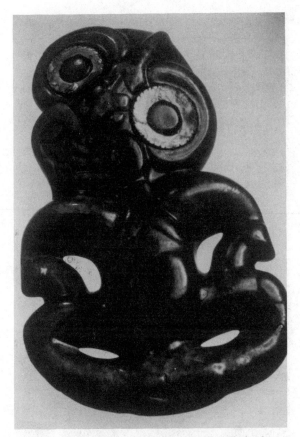

Figure 171. Maori Tiki figure, jade, New Zealand.

govern its destiny. As a result, there are innumerable depictions of Buddha, Krishna, and Christ. Places of worship are adorned with precious metals, beautiful carvings, paintings, mosaics, brilliant colors captured in glass—a far cry from prosaic art therapy, you may think.

And yet for those who search themselves through the art therapy process, there may be a similar use of images to connect with questions that extend beyond the finiteness of our own lives. The differences lie more in the nature of our society than in the art/spiritual/meaning process. No longer do we exist in a unified culture with a unified unquestioned formulation of the divine, peopled with significant personages and spirits. No longer do we know who we are in a fixed cosmos in which laws of life, death, transcendence, good fortune, and tragedy can be accounted for.

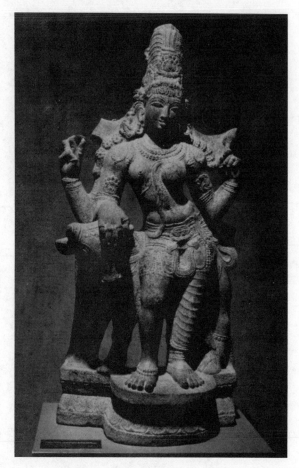

Figure 172. The god Shiva, India.

Even those of us who find solace within the teachings of a particular religious system are constantly being exposed to other points of view. It is on these shifting sands, rather than on the firmer footings of our ancestors' beliefs, that we attempt to build the meaning in our lives.

And what is the nature of these sands and the winds that drift them and the tides that wash over them? We live in memories of the holocaust, of the senseless slaughter in Vietnam. We live in the shadow of a nuclear arsenal that could destroy our entire civilization in 30 minutes. We have friends who have been raped. We have colleagues who work with violently and sexually abused children. We double lock our doors and cover

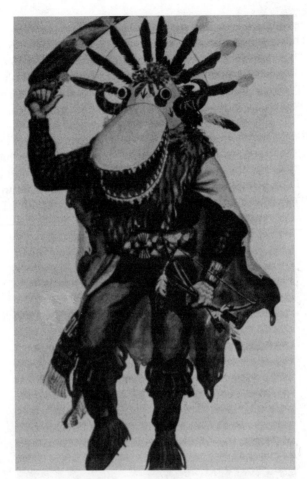

Figure 173. Hopi Indian ritual costume.

our jewelry when we ride the subway. We try to keep ourselves trim by resisting that extra helping of food at the same time the TV tells us of the widespread starvation in Africa. We live in a world beautiful beyond description where the air of Mexico City burns the eyes; mercury poisons the rivers and deforms babies born to their communities; death rains in acid from the skies; and here at the beach where I am writing the delicate balance of the ecology of the inland waterway is disrupted by the landfills for construction (I almost wrote "destruction" in an unintentional slip of the pen).

I'm sure you don't expect me to say that art therapy can save us from all this. There are artists and art therapists, however, who use the art therapy process to find themselves in this confusing world and to probe the meaning of their own existence through art-making. I have been a member of several groups in two cities who met for that purpose.

Many women have found spiritual meaning in the images and stories of goddesses or "the goddess" as embodiment of the earth or life. They have used art to deepen their connection with feminine aspects of birth, nurturing, creativity, and connection to the earth. Others have sought similar meanings without the goddess metaphor. One of the most powerful books I have read that connects the feminine with nature is Susan Griffin's *Woman and Nature, the Roaring Inside Her* (1978). This sort of

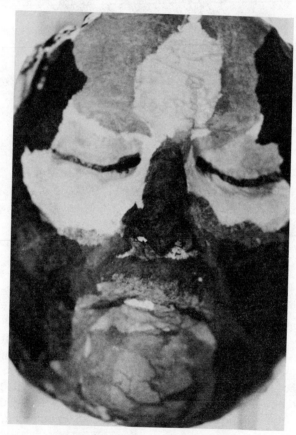

Figure 174. Interior of author's mask.

search is clearly a reaction to what is viewed as a destructive patriachal exploitation of nature compared to the reverence for nature characteristic of more "primitive" peoples and the creative harmony with natural forces that many believe is the only solution to our rapacious destruction of the land, sea, air, and living things around us.

Although women are seeking fuller and deeper identities in trying to create a place for themselves in today's world, the sort of "soul work" through art I am describing is by no means the special province of females. Nevertheless, as a profession composed primarily of women devoted to human healing, it is natural that art therapists examine their relationships to life through their art by looking to their female creativity as a source of unification. The separations many of us have felt as women—one from another, our minds from our bodies, our feelings from out intellect, women's present from women's history, humanity from the world of nature—are the splits women are trying to mend in a reunification on many levels. Art helps to forge these images.

Art therapy will not create ecological harmony any more than it will eliminate starvation and disease, end wars, or instigate loving human relationships. But the images created to "heal the soul" may help one to live in our less than perfect world.

The following are a few examples of my own sketches that touch on issues "beyond art therapy." I made a mask and colored it with tissue paper, both inside (Figure 174) and out (see Figure 169). I had intended the inside to be dark and the outside light, but more realistically, it did not work out that way. Almost without my conscious thought, the mask evoked the following poem:

MASQUE

If you want to find me
you must walk backward in the night
and look for me with closed eyes.
Still you will not see
the dark underside
of my eyelids
or hear the muffled murmers
bubbling in my throat.

If you want to see me
stare at the solstice sun's epiphany
until your eyes burn white
and your tears are scorched dry.

Still you will not feel my breath
stir the dark of its cool cave
and flutter the ashes
smoldering there.

If you want to know me
stand so still
your feet become roots in the ground
and your lips freeze
in the form of my name.
Then the moon will rain silver tears
upon the water
and my reflection will whisper in the waves:
"No one knows me."

Although the poem is about existential isolation, sharing it countered that feeling to some extent. It is in this way that the art therapy process can help us to reach both ourselves and others. Especially important to me in this poem was my unintentional merging of earth and body images. The connectedness reaches from my body to the earth to others—even in a poem about fundamental aloneness.

The Tarot is an ancient form of "divination" based on cards with evocative and sometimes cryptic pictures. Most who look to Tarot readings to inform their lives believe there is a purposefulness in the distribution of the cards. I enjoy giving Tarot readings, but I approach them somewhat differently. For me they are akin to the art therapy experience. Rather than employing their traditional meanings, I find that the cards' images stimulate my thinking in new and unexpected directions that are sometimes puzzling in juxtaposing disparate and seemingly unrelated elements in a single reading. Traveling these less likely paths often leads to new understandings. For some time I have wanted to create my own Tarot deck. Figure 175 is my sketch for the moon card. The crescent moon fills out to contain a foetus and drops gold and red sparks through the night sky to the ocean below. The image expresses the mysterious fecundity of life on earth and in the heavens. In the star card, Figure 176, a small figure stands on the edge of the earth and gazes in rapt wonder at a galaxy. The star's meaning for me embodies the immensity of the universe.

Some use art for modern day rituals of community celebration in which participants join together to share reverence for life and for each to explore his or her own spirit connections. Figure 177 was photographed at

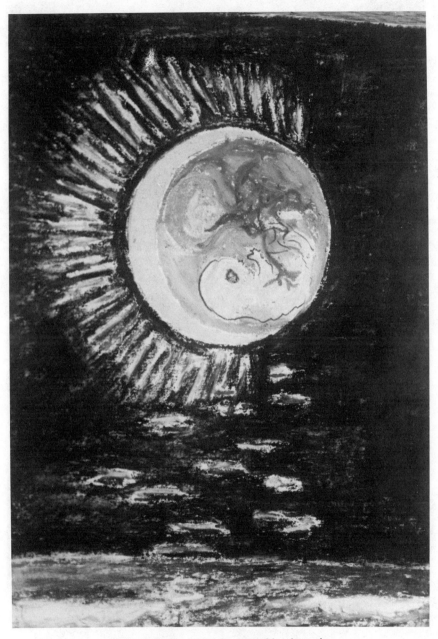

Figure 175. The Moon Tarot card by the author.

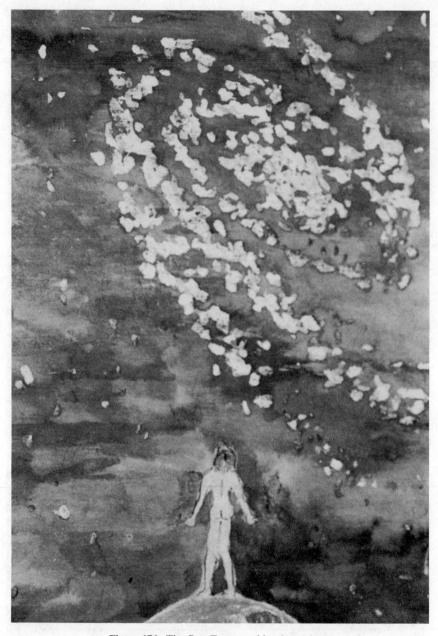

Figure 176. The Star Tarot card by the author.

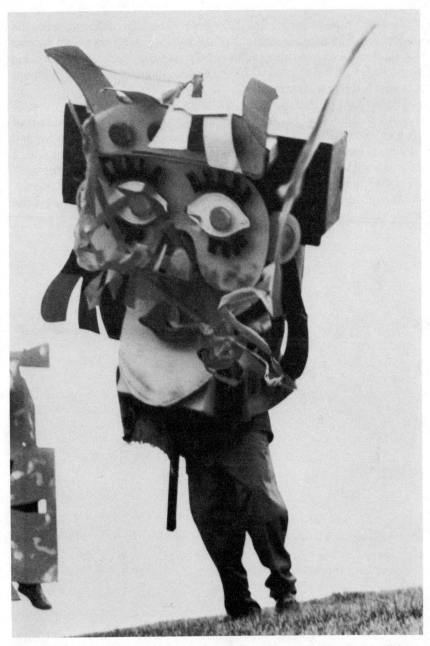

Figure 177. Oversize puppet in Big Fish Celebration Theatre autumn ritual in Chicago. (Photo courtesy of Stuart Abelson.)

an autumn ritual in which the hero enters the labyrinth and slays the dragon, in a ritualistic enactment of discovering one's own demons and slaying them. Prior to this enactment, the group prepared by undergoing many stages of the traditional hero journey, including creating the puppets and forming a labyrinth.

The content of therapy and spirituality merge in the human quest of creating meaning and in probing the fundamental existential questions of life and death. Ultimately, the art therapy process of creating images and relating to them leads to the sources of our own life energies. For those of us who wish to venture into these realms, our images illuminate the way. We create them; they create our world; our world creates us. We travel a spiral path with a beginning lost from sight and a destination beyond the bend, we know not how far.

Bibliography

Allen, P. & Wadeson, H. (1982). Art-making for conceptualization, integration, and self-awareness. In A. Evans (Ed.), *Art therapy: A bridge between worlds*. American Art Therapy Association Conference Proceedings, 1982.

American Psychiatric Association (1980). *Diagnostic and statistical manual of mental disorders (3rd ed.). DSM-III.* Washington, D.C.

Arnheim, R. (1969). *Visual thinking*. Berkeley: University of California Press.

Ault, R. (1977). Are you an artist or a therapist? A professional dilemma of art therapists. In R. Shoemaker and S. Gonick-Barris (Eds.), *Creativity and the art therapist's identity*. American Art Therapy Association Conference Proceedings, 1977.

Barron, F. (1968a). The dream of art and poetry. *Psychology Today*, 2:7.

Barron, F. (1968b). *Creativity and personal freedom*. Princeton, NJ: Van Nostrand.

Bruch, H. (1974). *Learning psychotherapy*. Cambridge, MA: Harvard University Press.

Chesler, P. (1972). *Women and Madness*. New York: Avon Books.

Cohen, F. (1985). *Incest markers in children's art work*. Presentation at Michigan Art Therapy Association Conference, 1985.

Dewald, P. (1971). *Psychotherapy: A dynamic approach*. New York: Basic Books.

Design for arts in education (1984). September/October, 86:1.

DiMaria, A. (1982). (Ed.), *Art therapy: Still growing*. American Art Therapy Association Conference Proceedings, 1982.

Edelson, M. (1963). *The termination of intensive psychotherapy*. Springfield, IL: Charles C. Thomas.

Goldenberg, N. (1979). *Changing of the gods*. Boston: Beacon Press.

Griffin, S. (1978). *Woman and nature, the roaring inside her*. New York: Harper & Row.

Guggenbuhl-Craig, A. (1971). *Power in the helping professions*. Zurich: Spring Publications.

Kellogg, R. (1969, 1970). *Understanding children's art*. Palo Alto, CA: Mayfield.

Kopp, S. (1972). *If you meet the buddha on the road, kill him*. Toronto: Bantam Books.

Kramer, E. (1971). *Art as therapy with children*. New York: Schocken Books.

Kramer, E. (1975). The problem of quality in art. In E. Ulman and P. Dachinger, (Eds.), *Art Therapy*. New York: Schocken Books.

Kramer, E. (1979). *Childhood and art therapy*. New York: Schocken Books.

Levinson, H. (1977). Termination of psychotherapy: Some salient issues. *Social Casework, 58*(8), 480–489.

Lowenfeld, V., & Brittain, W. L. (1970). *Creative and mental growth (5th ed.)*. New York: Macmillan.

Maslow, A. (1977). The creative attitude. In W. Anderson, (Ed.), *Theory and the arts: Tools of consciousness*. New York: Harper & Row.

McGee, T., Schuman, B., & Racusen, F. (1972). Termination in group psychotherapy. *American Journal of Psychotherapy. 26*(4), 521–532.

Moore, B., & Fine, B. (1968). *A Glossary of Psychoanalytic terms and concepts*. Washington, D.C.: American Psychiatric Association.

Moreno, G., & Wadeson, H. (1986). Art therapy for acculturation problems of hispanic clients. *Art Therapy, 3*, 122–130.

Naumburg, M. (1966). *Dynamically oriented art therapy: Its principles and practice*. New York: Grune & Stratton.

Reik, T. (1949). *Listening with the third ear*. New York: Farrar, Straus & Co.

Siden, N. (1985). Personal communication.

Sinrod, H. (1964). Communication through paintings in an art therapy group. *Bulletin of Art Therapy, 3*, 133–147.

Sullivan, H. S. (1940). *Conceptions of modern psychiatry*. New York: W. W. Norton.

Sullivan, H. S. (1953). *The interpersonal theory of psychiatry*. New York: W. W. Norton.

Wadeson, H. (1971a). Characteristics of art expression in depression. *Journal of Nervous and Mental Disease, 153*, 97–204.

Wadeson, H. (1971b). *Portraits of suicide*. Publication of exhibit, Annual Conference, American Psychiatric Association, 1971.

Wadeson, H. (1975). Suicide: Expression in images. *American Journal of Art Therapy, 14*, 75–82.

Wadeson, H. (1980). *Art Psychotherapy*. New York: John Wiley & Sons.

Wadeson, H. (1982a). The great debates. The place of art in art therapy: Speaking for the "art therapy position." In A. DiMaria (Ed.), *Art therapy: Still growing*. American Art Therapy Association Conference Proceedings, 1982.

Wadeson, H. (1982b). Where are our Ph.D.'s going? In L. Gantt (Ed.), *Focus on the future—the next ten years*. American Art Therapy Association Conference Proceedings, 1982.

Wadeson, H. & Carpenter, W. (1973). *Hallucinations and delusions*. Publication of exhibit, Annual Conference, American Psychiatric Association, 1973.

Wadeson, H., & Carpenter, W. (1974). Pictorial presentation of hallucinations and delusions. *Japanese Bulletin of Art Therapy, 5,* 97–104.

Wadeson, H., & Carpenter, W. (1976). Subjective experience of acute schizophrenia. *Schizophrenia Bulletin, 2,* 302–316.

Wadeson, H. & Fitzgerald, R. (1971). The marital relationship in manic-depressive illness: Conjoint psychiatric art evaluations. *Journal of Nervous and Mental Disease, 153,* 190–196.

Wohl, A., & Kaufman, B. (1985). *Silent screams and hidden cries.* New York: Brunner/Mazel.

Yalom, I. (1975). *The theory and practice of group psychotherapy.* New York: Basic Books.

Yalom, I. (1983). *In-patient group therapy.* New York: Basic Books.

Yalom, I., & Elkins, G. (1974). *Every day gets a little closer,* New York: Basic Books.

Author Index

Subject Index

Abstract pictures, 81
Acceptance of patient, 57
Acculturation problems, 219–223
Acting out behavior reflecting anxiety, 206–207
Activity therapy, 238
Adolescent patients, 62, 171, 173
Alcoholism, 93, 100
Ambiguity:
    in title "art therapist," 20
    tolerance for, in creative people, 17–18
American Art Therapy Association, 33, 240, 251, 252, 273
    Guidelines for Education and Training, 33, 273
Anger, therapist's, 118
Anxiety:
    case example reflected in acting-out behavior, 206–207
    of patient, 60–61
    of therapist, 17, 126
Apathy, 82
Art, as therapy, 159, 235, 259–271
    case example using insight-oriented art therapy, 260–263
    with children, 264–265
    "pursuit of image," 265–270
Art activities, 27, 31, 65
Art classes, development of art therapy, 20
Art club, noninsight oriented groups, 163–164
Art competition, in group art therapy, 144
Art displays, 62
Art education, 19

Art experience, factor in group art therapy, 153
Art exploration process, 25
Art expression:
    of art therapist, 12, 179, 260, 280
    art therapist's reaction to, 179
    encouragement and exploration, 109
    in group art therapy, 141, 144, 147, 148
    historical use, 294–295
    media choice, 70
    of patient, 21, 23, 26, 57, 62, 63, 65, 84, 90, 93, 105
    psychic interior, 99
    of psychotically depressed patients, 61
    relating to schizophrenics, 128–130
    roadblocks, 56–65, 179
    understanding, 67
    vehicle in terminating treatment, 194
Art instruction, 39
Artist, 21
    art therapist as, 18–21
Artistic accomplishment, 57
Artistic alphabet, 99
Artistic excellence, 173
Artistic merit:
    of art therapist's art, 12
    of patient's art, 62, 259
Artistic skill, of patient, 42, 144
Artistic style, of patient, 113
Art-making, 1, 2, 7, 25, 26, 30–31, 40, 65, 82–84, 260
    of art therapist, 12, 19–20, 194, 298
    with clients, 133–137, 194
    as extraordinary skill, case study, 204

311